Health For All
Towards the 21st Century

英語で読む
21世紀の
健康

阿部裕子
正木美知子

    People living in developed countries today have the opportunity to be healthier than ever before. Our understanding of how the body works has broadened rapidly in the last few years, paralleled by equally dramatic improvements in medical technology. As a result of this progress, a person's chances of staying healthy into old age depend increasingly on following expert advice on a healthy life-style, making full use of preventive techniques such as vaccination and screening tests, and seeking medical advice from your physician at the first sign of illness.
    Today, most children in developed countries are healthier than ever before; a majority can expect to live well beyond the age of 70. These achievements are partly due to improvements in public health, such as the provision of safe water supplies and sewage disposal systems, adequate housing, and good nutrition, and partly to improvements in medical care.

講談社サイエンティフィク

出 典 一 覧

A   Charles B. Clayman *et al.*, *The American Medical Association Encyclopedia of Medicine*, Random House (1989)
B   Annette Spence, *Encyclopedia of Good Health: Substance Abuse*, Mario Orlandi & Donald Prue (series ed.), Michael Friedman Publishing Group, Inc. (1989)
C   *Women and Tobacco*, WHO (1992)
D   *The UNAIDS Report*, The Joint United Nations Programme on HIV/AIDS (1999)
E   The Global Plague of AIDS, Weekly Review, *The New York Times*, Apr. 23 (2000)
       Copyright©2000 by the New York Times Co. Reprinted by permission.
F   Annette Spence, *Encyclopedia of Good Health: Nutrition*, Mario Orlandi & Donald Prue (series ed.) Michael Friedman Publishing Group, Inc. (1989)
G   Young Japanese men losing war on weight, *Daily Yomiuri*, Feb. 27 (2000)
H   *Obesity*, WHO (1998)
I   Annette Spence, *Encyclopedia of Good Health: Exercise*, Mario Orlandi & Donald Prue (series editors) Michael Friedman Publishing Group, Inc. (1989)
J   Gert Lynge Sorensen, *Equal Opportunities for Disabled Persons — the Danish Way*, Danish Export Group Association (1994)
K   Wheelchair Etiquette, excerpt from *"What do I do when I meet a person in a wheelchair?"*, National Easter Seal Society
L   *The World Health Report 1999*, WHO (1999)

URL①   http://health.yahoo.com/health/diet/healthy_diet_1.html
URL②   http://health.yahoo.com/health/diet/healthy_diet_2.html
URL③   http://health.yahoo.com/health/Diseases_and_Conditions/Disease_Feed_Data/Physical_activity/index.html
URL④   http://health.yahoo.com/health/Diseases_and_Conditions/Disease_Feed_Data/Keeping_fit/
URL⑤   http://aging.ufl.edu/apadiv20/vili4.htm
URL⑥   http://aging.ufl.edu/apadiv20/vili5.htm
URL⑦   http://www.atmeda.org/whatis/whitepaper.html

        NIAAA: National Institute on Alcohol Abuse and Alcoholism
        USDA: United States Department of Agriculture
        Ministry of Health and Welfare: 厚生省

　テキストとして採用した英文は，世界共通語としての英語の現状をそのままに反映して，多様性を示しているが，書き手の意向を尊重して，用語，文法はそのままとした．ただ，学習者の混乱を最小限にとどめるため，つづりはアメリカ英語の表記法に統一した．

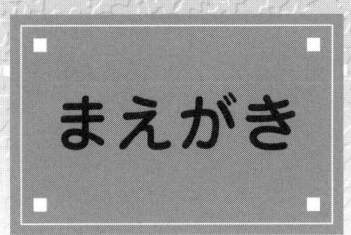

　21世紀の特徴として予測されうることの中には，次の2点を含むことができるでしょう．ひとつには，医学を含む科学技術のとどまることのない発展であり，もうひとつは，人類がその種としての進化の歴史上いまだかって経験したことのない多くの個体数をもって，この地球上で生存していかなければならないという人類の棲息条件の変化です．世界の人口は20世紀中に60億人，2025年には80億人を超えると推計されています．

　私たちの健康は，個人レベルでは，ひとりひとりの人生のあり方─生活の質─に深くかかわってくる問題を提起します．他方，社会レベルにおいては，地球という限定された空間の与える環境の中で，多数の人間が最大限に快適に共存する方法をいかにして見いだすか，という課題を提起します．

　この問題解決を目的として，人類が20世紀の半ばに考案した制度が，世界保健機関（WHO）です．WHOが発信する膨大なメッセージの中で，今，現在の地球上で，人類の健康にかかわるいろいろな問題をどのように認識し，それにどう対処していくべきなのか，とくに，若い人たちに知ってほしいと願うものを選んで，それを中心にしてこの教科書が出来上がりました．

　この本は，英語教科の教科書としては，「意味のある内容を学びながら，それを伝える手段としての英語を使う力をのばすこと─content-based, communicative language learning」を目的としています．

　本書の完成のために，英文資料の教育的目的への利用に御理解を示して下さった各位に感謝いたします．医学全般について御教示いただいた三木雪子氏，英語に関する貴重なアドバイスをいただいたRonald Cline, Jenine Heaton両氏，栄養学の分野において御協力いただいた四谷美和子氏に厚くお礼申し上げます．また，講談社サイエンティフィクの吉田茂子出版部長の終始かわらぬ御鞭撻がなければ本書は完成しなかったことと思います．深く感謝いたします．本書の作成にあたりましては，最善を尽くしたつもりですが，まだまだ不備な点があることと思います．各位からの御指導をいただければ幸いです．

　2000年7月

阿部　祚子
正木美知子

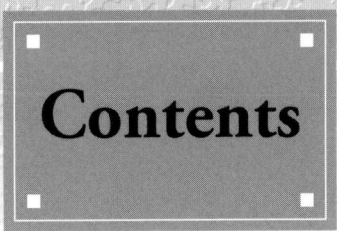

出典一覧　　ii
まえがき　　iii

Chapter 1 : Introduction　　はじめに
    I.　What Is the World Health Organization?　………　WHOとは?　………………………… 1
    II.　Staying Healthy　………………………………………　健康であること　……………………… 5

Chapter 2 : Tobacco Smoking　　喫煙
    I.　Smoke : What's in There?　………………………　タバコの煙：中には何が?　………… 10
    II.　Women and Tobacco Use　………………………　女性と喫煙　…………………………… 15

Chapter 3 : Alcohol　　飲酒
    I.　How Alcohol Acts on the Body　………………　お酒を飲んだらどうなるの?　……… 20
    II.　Drinking in Moderation　…………………………　ほどほどに飲みましょう　…………… 25

Chapter 4 : HIV/AIDS　　HIVとエイズ
    I.　What Is AIDS?　………………………………………　エイズってどんな病気?　…………… 30
    II.　The Global Plague of AIDS　……………………　エイズの世界的な広がり　…………… 34

Chapter 5 : Nutrition　　栄養
    I.　Diet Is Important to Health　……………………　食事は健康にとってたいせつなもの … 40
    II.　Food Guide Pyramid　………………………………　フードガイドピラミッド　…………… 44

Contents

Chapter 6 : Obesity   肥満
    I. Why Do People Get Fat? .... 肥満とは？ 49
    II. Indices of Overweight .... 肥満をはかる指数 54

Chapter 7 : Exercise   運動
    I. Physical Activity and the Use of Calories .... 身体活動とエネルギー消費 59
    II. Guidelines for Exercise .... よい運動のためのガイドライン 64

Chapter 8 : Disabilities   障害
    I. Where There's a Will, There's a Way .... 意志あるところ，道あり 68
    II. Accessibility for All for the New Millennium ...... 新ミレニアムに向けて，すべての人のためにアクセサビリティを 73

Chapter 9 : Aging   高齢化
    I. Population Aging — A Public Challenge .... 高齢化—社会への挑戦 78
    II. Adult Development and Aging .... 能力開発と高齢化 83

Chapter 10 : Health Agenda for the 21st Century   21世紀への健康課題
    I. Health Agenda for the 21st Century 21世紀への健康課題 88
    II. Global Health Care System
        — Health in the Digital Age .... デジタル時代がもたらすもの 92

Chapter 1
Introduction

はじめに

I. What Is the World Health Organization (WHO)?

WHOとは？

FACTS *

1830	Cholera <u>overruns</u> Europe
1851	First International Sanitary Conference is held in Paris to produce an <u>international sanitary convention</u>, but fails.
1945	United Nations Conference on International Organization in San Francisco <u>unanimously</u> approves a proposal by Brazil and China to establish a new, <u>autonomous</u>, international health organization.
1948	WHO <u>Constitution</u> <u>comes into force</u> on 7 April (now marked as World Health Day each year), when the 26th of the 61 Member States who signed it <u>ratified</u> its signature. Later, the First World Health <u>Assembly</u> is held in Geneva with <u>delegations</u> from 53 governments that by then were Members. [WHO]

＊歴史年表では過去の出来事でも現在形の時制を用いて記述します．

Notes　overrun：猛威をふるう　international sanitary convention：国際公衆衛生協定

unanimously：全会一致で　autonomous：独立した，自律的な　constitution：憲章　come into force：発効する　ratify：批准する　assembly：総会　delegation：代表団

■■ Pre-reading activities

1. FACTSを読んで次の質問に英語で答えなさい．

    (1) What does WHO stand for?

    (2) When was the first international conference on health issues held in Paris?

    (3) How many Member States had signed the WHO Constitution by 7 April, 1948?

    (4) How many Member States does WHO have at present?

■■ Read the passage

　　WHO stands for the World Health Organization. Founded in 1948, the World Health Organization is a specialized agency of the United Nations with 191* Member States. All countries which are Members of the United Nations may become members of WHO by accepting its Constitution. Other countries may be admitted as members when their applications have been approved by a simple majority vote of the World Health Assembly. It leads the world alliance for Health for All.

　　WHO promotes technical cooperation for health among nations, carries out programs to control and eradicate disease and strives to improve the quality of human life.

　　WHO has four main functions:
    1. to give worldwide guidance in the field of health
    2. to set global standards for health
    3. to cooperate with governments in strengthening national health programmes

4. to develop and <u>transfer</u> appropriate health technology, information and standards.

Notes agency：機関　admitted：加盟が認められる　application：加盟の申請　majority vote：投票による単純多数決　the World Health Assembly：世界保健機関の総会　alliance：同盟　program：計画　eradicate：根絶させる　global standards：全世界に共通の基準　transfer：普及させる　＊2000年現在

Post-reading activities

1. 次の英文のうち，内容が正しいものにはT，間違っているものにはFを（　）に記入しなさい．

    (1) The World Health Organization is an agency of the United Nations. （　）

    (2) To be admitted as a member of WHO, a nation needs to be a Member of the United Nations. （　）

    (3) WHO promotes technical cooperation for health among nations, but does not engage in any programs to eradicate disease. （　）

    (4) WHO has five main functions. （　）

世界の国々の分類

国連では，世界の国々を多角的な指標に基づいて，発展の4段階に分けて分類しています．WHOも種々の統計にこの分類を用いています．

1. Least developed countries：Afghanistan, Ethiopia, Ugandaなど
2. Developing countries — excluding least developed countries：Algeria, Brazil, Philippines, Peru, Thailandなど
3. Economies in transition：Albania, Czech Republic, Russian Federationなど
4. Developed market economies：Australia, France, Germany, Japan, USAなど

この分類は絶対的なものではなく，年ごとに分類の見直しがおこなわれます．

1 : Introduction

2. WHOの加盟国は世界6地域におかれた事務局の管轄下におかれています．次の加盟国はどの地域に属するでしょうか．

> Albania, Algeria, Argentina, Australia, Austria, Bangladesh, Barbados, Belgium, Benin, Bolivia, Brazil, Chile, China, Croatia, Cuba, Cyprus, Jamaica, Japan, Jordan, Kenya, Kuwait, Netherlands, Nicaragua, Nigeria, Norway, Papua New Guinea, Republic of Korea, South Africa, Spain, Thailand, United States of America

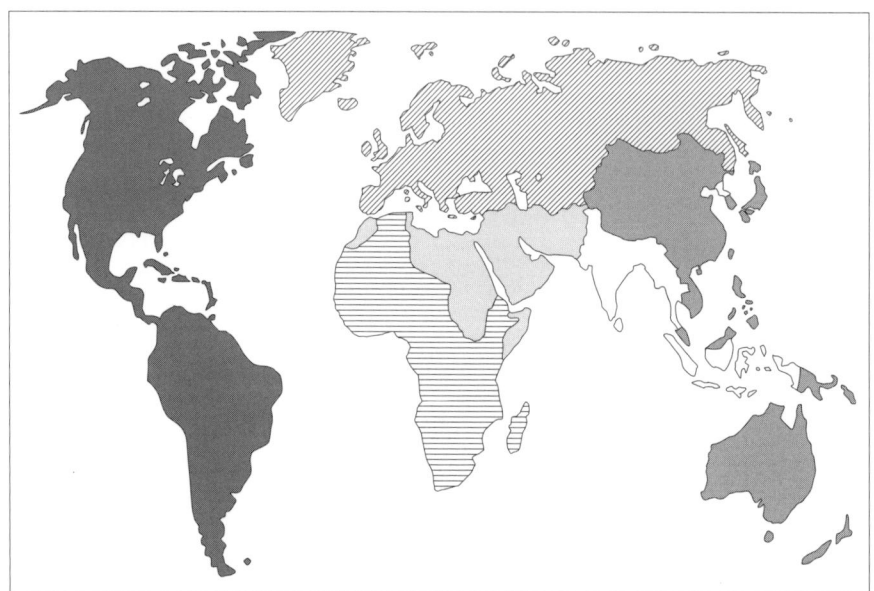

Regional Office for Africa: Benin, Kenya, Nigeria, South Africa

Regional Office for the Americas: Argentina, Barbados, Bolivia, Brazil, Chile, Cuba, Jamaica, Nicaragua, United States of America

Regional Office for South-East Asia: Bangladesh, Thailand

Regional Office for Europe: Albania, Austria, Belgium, Croatia, Cyprus, Netherlands, Norway, Spain

Regional Office for the Eastern Mediterranean: Algeria, Jordan, Kuwait

Regional Office for the Western Pacific: Australia, China, Japan, Papua New Guinea, Republic of Korea

II. Staying Healthy

健康であること

> **WHO Definition of Health**
>
> Health is a state of complete physical, mental, and scocial well-being and not merely the absence of disease or infirmity.

Notes　well-being：望ましい状態にあること　infirmity：虚弱であること

▎Pre-reading activities

1. 上のWHOの「健康」の定義に含まれるそれぞれの項目について，あなたの現状を書きましょう．

   Physical well-being:

   Mental well-being:

   Social well-being:

2. 次の21世紀の健康に関する質問に，あなた自身の予測を○で囲みなさい．
   (1) Will the world continue to grow healthier?　　Yes　　No
   (2) If populations live longer, will these extra years be healthy and productive?　Yes　　No
   (3) Will we conquer the common cold?　　Yes　　No
   (4) Will deaths from cancer begin to decline?　　Yes　　No
   (5) Will the gaps between the health of rich and poor grow ever wider?　Yes　　No

Read the passage

下の文を読んで，現代に生きる私たちの健康についての一般的な概観をつかみましょう．

Staying healthy

People living in developed countries today have the opportunity to be healthier than ever before. Our understanding of how the body works has broadened rapidly in the last few years, <u>paralleled by</u> equally dramatic improvements in medical technology. As a result of this progress, a person's chances of staying healthy into old age depend increasingly on following expert advice on a healthy life-style, making full use of <u>preventive techniques</u> such as <u>vaccination</u> and <u>screening tests</u>, and seeking medical advice from your <u>physician</u> at the first sign of illness.

Today, most children in developed countries are healthier than ever before; a majority can expect to live well beyond the age of 70. These achievements are partly due to improvements in public health, such as the provision of safe water supplies and <u>sewage disposal systems</u>, adequate housing, and good nutrition, and partly to improvements in medical care.

The health of women today can be carefully monitored before and during pregnancy, and during the birth of the baby. After birth, the newborn infant is closely examined and, if necessary, provided with <u>specialized care</u>.

Throughout infancy and childhood, children are <u>immunized</u> against <u>infections</u> and given vision and hearing tests, as well as tests for physical and mental development. As a result, any <u>problems</u> can be detected and treated promptly.

In the US and Europe, the principal causes of death or disability in youth and middle age are preventable. In early adult life, most deaths are due to accidents or violence; other important causes include suicide, and <u>complications</u> of <u>drug abuse</u> and sexual habits (notably by HIV/AIDS). In addition, the risk of developing the principal serious disorders of middle age—<u>coronary heart disease</u> and cancer—is reduced by following a healthy life-style and avoiding known health hazards, especially tobacco and alcohol.

Avoiding premature death is not the only benefit to be gained from following a healthy life-style. The quality of life can also improve: the body's natural aging processes are slowed, and physical and mental vigor are retained for much longer.

〔出典 A. p.16, L1〜11, p.17, L1〜19, R1〜8, R24〜28〕

Notes　paralleled by〜：〜とあいまって　preventive technique：予防的医療技術　vaccination：予防接種　screening tests：スクリーニング(検査，選別)　physician：内科医　sewage disposal system：下水処理システム　specialized care：専門医によるケア　immunize：免疫をつける　infection：感染症　problems：広義の病気の意味でよく使われる　complications：合併症　drug abuse：薬物乱用　coronary heart disease：冠動脈性心臓病　health hazards：健康への害　premature death：早死に，早世　physical and mental vigor：体力と気力

■ Post-reading activities

1. ＿＿＿に入る最も適切なものをa〜cから選びなさい．

    (1) People living in ＿＿＿ countries today have the opportunity to be healthier than ever.
        a. developing
        b. developed
        c. least developed

    (2) Today a majority of children in developed countries expect to live well beyond ＿＿＿ .
        a. 40
        b. 50
        c. 70

    (3) The risk of women in developed countries dying in childbirth has ＿＿＿ .
        a. increased
        b. declined
        c. doubled

    (4) Throughout infancy and childhood, children are immunized against ＿＿＿ .

1 : Introduction

   a. coronary heart disease
   b. complications
   c. infections
(5) Immunization is an effective _____ .
   a. monitoring device
   b. preventive technique
   c. provision of safe water
(6) By following a healthy life-style, one is likely to _____ .
   a. stay healthy into old age
   b. die prematurely in youth
   c. become bedridden in middle age

2. 次の(　)に入れる適切な語句を下の枠内から選びなさい.
   (1) Our understanding of how the body works has (　　).
   (2) Safe water supplies are not available in every (　　) country.
   (3) (　　) women should be monitored carefully for health problems.
   (4) Immunization of a children can save many lives from (　　).
   (5) HIV/AIDS is a preventable (　　).
   (6) The risk of (　　) coronary disease and cancer can be reduced.
   (7) The (　　) of life is determined by a person's life-style.
   (8) Improvements in (　　) have contributed a great deal to creating healthier environments.

   | disease | public health | developing | broadened | pregnant |
   | quality | premature death | infections | | |

3. 次の英文が本文の内容にあっていればT, 間違っていればFを(　)に記入しなさい.
   (1) A person's chance of staying healthy into old age depends on how much money he or she has. (　　)
   (2) Improvements in medical care are partly responsible for the achievement of a longer, healthier life. (　　)

(3) All diseases can be prevented by following a healthy life-style. (　)

(4) In developed countries, the principal causes of death in youth are accidents or violence. (　)

(5) Knowledge about our bodies has played a key role in making our lives longer and healthier. (　)

お元気ですか？―QOLとDALE

元気ってなんでしょうか．WHOがかかげる「健康」の定義では，健康とはただ病気でない状態をいうのではなく，心身がともに健康な状態で社会生活を送れることを意味します．つまり元気でいきいき暮らせることです．これは，Quality of Life（QOL）―「生活の質」をも取り入れた考え方です．

健康で長生きできることは，誰もが望むことです．そこで，この状態をあらわすために，Healthy Life Expectancy―「健康寿命」という考えがうまれました．この算定に用いられるのが，Disability Adjusted Life Expectancy（DALE）―「障害期間調整後の平均余命」です．種々の障害，疾病をQOLにおよぼす影響の程度に応じて重み付けをして数量化して年数（DALY, p.39参照）であらわし，Total Health Expectancy平均寿命（平均余命）から差し引きます．これによって，病気，事故などによる障害を，ただ死亡の原因としてだけでなく，それが人の一生におよぼす影響の大きさという視点から見ることができます．病気，事故などによる障害が，元気で長生きできるはずの人生からむざむざと何年間を奪い取ってしまうか（Disease Burden―「疾病負担」）によって，国民全体など「集団」の健康度をあらわす指標として用いられます．

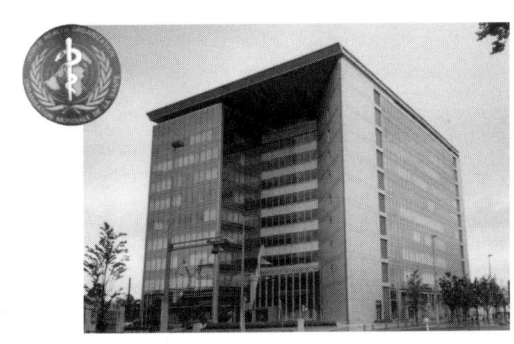

IHD（国際健康開発）センタービルにWHO健康開発総合研究センターがある（神戸市）

WHOに加盟している192か国の中で，この「健康寿命」の最長寿国は，日本の74.5歳で，これは最短国との間に26歳もの開きがあります．2位以下は，オーストラリア（73.2），フランス（73.1），スウェーデン（73.0），スペイン（72.8），イタリア（72.7），ギリシャ（72.5），モナコ（72.4），アンドラ（72.3）と続きます．（*The World Health Report 2000*, WHOによる）

Chapter 2
Tobacco Smoking

喫煙

I. Smoke: What's in There?

タバコの煙：中には何が？

> That nicotine is used as a weed killer? It's a poison. Sixty milligrams of nicotine taken at one time will kill that average adult human being by <u>paralyzing</u> breathing. The reason it does not kill smokers quickly is that they <u>inhale</u> tiny <u>doses</u> (a cigarette has between 0.5 and 2 milligrams), which are quickly used or <u>disposed of</u> by the body.

Notes   paralyze：麻痺させる   inhale：吸い込む   dose：服用量   dispose of：処理する

■ Pre-reading activities

1. How many respiration organs does inhaled cigarette smoke affect?
   タバコを吸った時，その煙はどの器官に触れることになるのでしょうか．枠内にその器官の名前が英語で記してあります．それぞれどこにあるのか絵に書き込みなさい．

   | bronchi | throat | mouth | bronchioles | windpipe | lungs |

I. Smoke: What's in There?

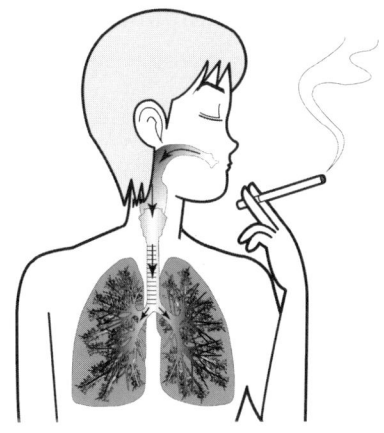
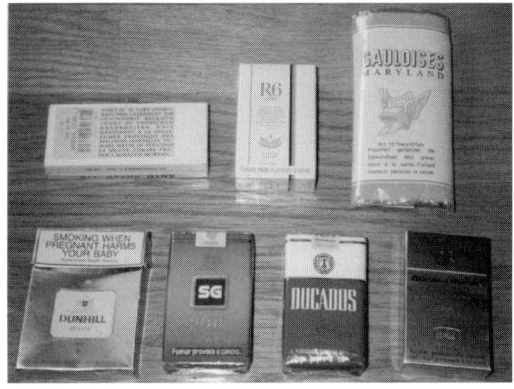

2. (　　)の中に入る最も適切なものをa〜dから選びなさい．

(1) Eventually, he overcame his cigarette (　　).
　　a. inhaling　　b. drinking　　c. addiction　　d. smoke

(2) Tobacco contains a lot of (　　).
　　a. carcinogens　　b. fluid　　c. nutrients　　d. minerals

(3) Tobacco smoking may cause (　　) diseases.
　　a. respiratory　　b. digestive　　c. mental
　　d. communicable

(4) Sixty milligrams of nicotine taken at a time is (　　).
　　a. allowed　　b. accepted　　c. appropriate　　d. fatal

Read the passage

タバコはどうして体に悪いのでしょうか．以下の英文を読んでみましょう．

　タバコの煙は何千という化学物質からなっていますが，体に最も悪い影響をあたえるものは，ニコチン，タール，そして一酸化炭素です．

Smoke: What's in there?

　Tobacco smoke is not just smoke: Scientists can break it down into thousands of chemicals and <u>particles</u>. Basically, however, most effects of tobacco smoke are related to three major components.

Nicotine

　The colorless, oily chemical in tobacco, is responsible for cigarette <u>addiction</u>. It races from the lungs to the bloodstream to the brain in seconds to stimulate the heart and nervous system. When the body gets used to having a certain level of nicotine in the bloodstream, victims become physically dependent. Not only does this "drug" work on the brain, it also reduces the amount of blood carried to the heart, which eventually damages the heart tissues. Nicotine also affects the digestive system.

Tar

Tar is the brownish, sticky stuff you see on ashtrays. Produced when tobacco is burned, tar is made of several hundred different chemicals, many of them <u>carcinogens</u>, which means they cause or help cause cancer. When smoke is inhaled, tar gets trapped in the lungs, and —just as it sticks to an ashtray—coats the <u>respiratory</u> (breathing) <u>tract</u>. This physical contact with tar promotes cancer. Tar can also damage the lungs' <u>mucus</u> (body fluid) and <u>cilia</u> (little hairline structures) that help sweep out <u>foreign materials</u>.

Carbon Monoxide

Carbon monoxide is the same gas that comes out of a car's <u>exhaust pipe</u>. As you know, breathing these fumes can be <u>fatal</u>, so it makes sense that inhaling carbon monoxide in cigarette smoke is also dangerous. (Cigarette smokers have up to ten times as much carbon monoxide in their blood as nonsmokers.) When carbon monoxide enters the bloodstream from a cigarette, it prevents some of the <u>blood cells</u> from carrying oxygen to parts of the body. This is why smokers are often short of breath, their muscles hurt, and their endurance suffers during exercise. Carbon monoxide also damages <u>blood vessels</u> and eyesight.

［出典 B. p.25 全文］

Notes　　particles：粒子　addiction：中毒　carcinogen：発がん物質　respiratory tract：気道　mucus：粘液　cilia：繊毛　foreign materials：異物　exhaust pipe：排気筒　fatal：命にかかわる　blood cells：血球　blood vessels：血管

"A pack-of-a-day smoker pours
a cup of tar into his lungs each year."

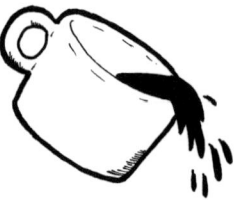

I. Smoke: What's in There?

▪▪ Post-reading activities

1. ＿＿に入る最も適切なものをa〜cから選びなさい.

    (1) Tobacco smoke is made up of ＿＿＿＿ .
        a. smoke like any other smoke
        b. thousands of chemicals and particles
        c. three major components

    (2) What is responsible for cigarette addiction is ＿＿＿＿ .
        a. nicotine
        b. tar
        c. carbon monoxide

    (3) Tar is made of several hundred different chemicals which ＿＿＿＿ .
        a. reduce the amount of blood carried to the heart
        b. damage the heart tissue
        c. cause or help cause cancer

    (4) Smokers are often short of breath, their muscles hurt, and their endurance suffers during exercise because ＿＿＿＿ .
        a. they are addicted to tobacco
        b. tar can damage the lungs' mucus and cilia that help sweep out foreign materials
        c. carbon monoxide prevents some of the blood cells from carrying oxygen to the parts of the body

2. passageにでてきた表現を使って次の文を英訳しなさい.

    (1) 化粧品(cosmetics)はさまざまな化学物質に分析することができます.
        break〜down into：細かく分析(分類)する

    (2) 私はその壊れた窓ガラスに責任はありません.
        be responsible for〜：〜に責任がある

    (3) タバコを子どもたちの前では吸わないということは道理にかなっています.
        It makes sense that〜：〜は道理にかなっている

3. 次のグラフは日本の喫煙率，タバコ消費量，年齢による調整を行った肺がんの死亡率を表しています．英文が，グラフと一致すればTを，一致しなければFを（　）に記入しなさい．

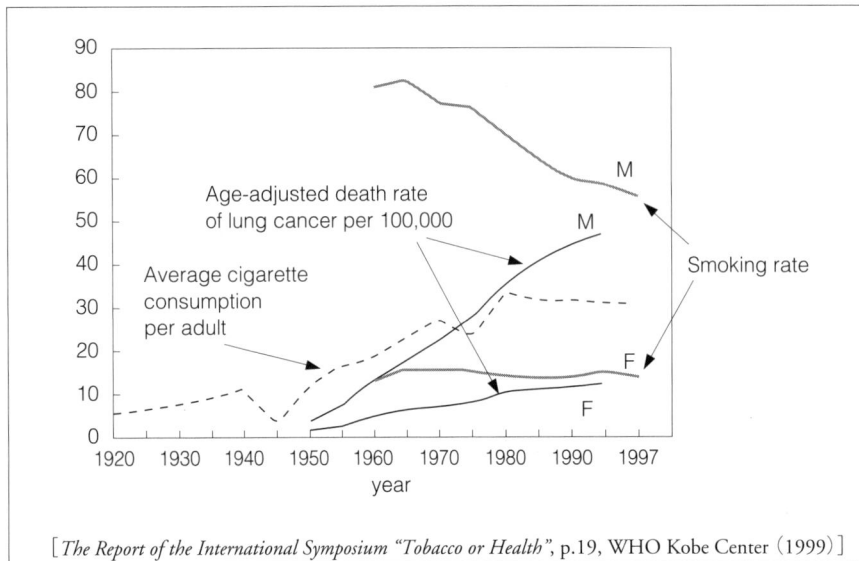

Trends in the smoking rate, cigarette consumption and the age-adjusted death rate of lung cancer in Japan
source: Japan Tobacco Indust. Inc. and Vital Statistics of Japan

[*The Report of the International Symposium "Tobacco or Health"*, p.19, WHO Kobe Center (1999)]

(1) Although the smoking rate in Japan has been declining gradually in recent years, the rate for adult males is still high. (　)

(2) The smoking rate for adult females has remained relatively low. (　)

(3) The age-adjusted death rate of lung cancer per 100,000 is declining for both sexes. (　)

(4) Average cigarette consumption per adult has been decreasing. (　)

(5) Though the smoking rate is rising, the risk of lung cancer is decreasing. (　)

(6) In the past 32 years, the smoking rate has declined by 27.9 % for females and by 4.4 % for males. (　)

II. Women and Tobacco Use

女性と喫煙

FACTS

Use of tobacco is a contributory factor in about 90 % of cases of lung cancer, over 80 % of cases of chronic bronchitis and emphysema, and 20-25 % of deaths from coronary heart disease and stroke. Altogether, smoking is estimated to kill approximately 3 million people each year. At present, fewer than 20 % of these deaths are among women, but as more and more women in both developed and developing countries starts to adopt patterns of smoking previously seen mainly in men, this proportion is likely to increase dramatically.   [WHO]

Notes　contributory：一因となる　lung cancer：肺がん　chronic：慢性の　bronchitis：気管支炎　emphysema：気腫　coronary heart disease：冠動脈性心臓病　stroke：卒中　altogether：全体で　developed countries：先進国　developing countries：発展途上国

■ Pre-reading activities

1. グラフは1957年から1987年までの男女別の肺がんの死亡率の推移です．1957年の男女別の死亡率を100として表されています．英文はこのグラフの説明です．（　）の中から文中の語として最も適切なものを選びなさい．

　　Since the 1960s, there has been a (a. steady and dramatic　b. steady and slight　c. steady and slow) increase in the number of deaths from lung cancer among women; overall, the death rate from lung cancer among women in developed countries has increased by almost (a. 100 %　b. 200 %　c. 300 %). It has (a. caught up with　b. fallen far short of　c. surpassed) the relative lung cancer mortality among men.

2 : Tobacco Smoking

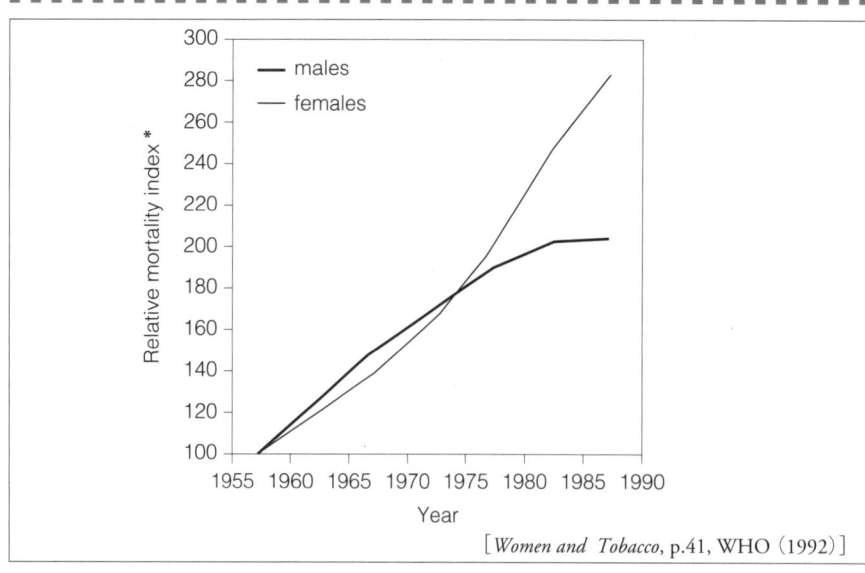

Trends in lung cancer mortality by sex in developed countries, 1957-87

*Death rate for each period expressed as a percentage of the mortality level for 1955-59

[*Women and Tobacco*, p.41, WHO (1992)]

2. (　)の中に入る最も適切なものをa～dから選びなさい．
  (1) The WHO survey showed a higher (　) of smoking among young women than young men in some countries.
    a. duration　　b. mortality　　c. prevalence
    d. preference
  (2) It was (　) that he was ill.
    a. apparent　　b. appear　　c. doubt　　d. seems
  (3) In developed countries, smoking by women used to be socially (　).
    a. acceptable　　b. unacceptable　　c. admitted
    d. prohibited
  (4) (　) tobacco marketing encourages young people to smoke.
    a. positive　　b. negative　　c. obscure　　d. aggressive

∷Read the passage

　世界的にみて，男性の喫煙率は総じて減ってきていますが，女性の喫煙率は総じて増えてきています．WHOはこの問題を先進国と発展途上国とにわけて事情を探っています．

　Tobacco is the single largest cause of <u>premature adult death</u> throughout the world. Over the next 30 years tobacco-related deaths among women will be more than double, so that by the year 2020 well over a million adult women will die every year from tobacco-related illnesses. Currently, in the developed world, the prevalence of smoking among women is approximately 20-35 %, whereas in the developing world, it is estimated at 2-10 %.

In the developed countries, smoking by women was socially unacceptable for many years. However, by the mid-20th century, in most developed countries, smoking by women had increased rapidly. As the health hazards of tobacco became apparent, the prevalence of smoking among men declined in some developed countries. Prevalence rates among women did not begin to decline until later and then only in a few countries; the two rates are currently converging in several countries. Today, in many developed countries, smoking is predominantly a practice of young women, women with limited education, and women of low socioeconomic status.

In the past, cultural norms were a powerful deterrent to women's smoking in the developing world, although there have always been areas in which women have practiced traditional forms of tobacco use. Currently, in the developing world smoking is linked with a cosmopolitan and affluent life-style. With increasing urbanization and career-oriented education, and increasing spending power, many young women who aspire to this life-style have taken up smoking. There is grave concern that these aspirations, fuelled by aggressive tobacco marketing, will result in increased prevalence rates among women in developing countries, further compounding their present difficulties. 〔出典 C. p.3, l. 1～25〕

Notes premature adult death：成人の早死に prevalence：普及，ここでは喫煙率 approximately：約，およそ health hazards：健康への害 apparent：明らかな converge：収束する predominantly：圧倒的に cultural norms：文化規範 deterrent：抑止力 cosmopolitan：国際的な urbanization：都市化 aggressive：攻撃的な compound：度合いを増す

▪ Post-reading activities

1. ＿＿＿に入る最も適切なものをa～cから選びなさい．

(1) Over the next 30 years tobacco-related deaths among women

will be more than double, so that by the year 2020 _____.
   a. tobacco-related illnesses will prevail
   b. tobacco will kill more than a million adult women
   c. less than a million adult women will die every year from tobacco-related illnesses

(2) By the mid-20th century, in most developed countries, smoking by women _____.
   a. had increased dramatically
   b. had decreased rapidly
   c. had remained almost the same

(3) As the health hazards of tobacco became apparent, _____.
   a. the prevalence of smoking among women declined in some developed countries
   b. the prevalence of smoking among both men and women declined in some developed countries
   c. the smoking rate among men decreased in some developed countries

(4) Today, in many developed countries, young women _____.
   a. smoke more than young men
   b. do not like smoking
   c. predominantly practice smoking

(5) In the past, smoking was discouraged among women because _____.
   a. smoking was linked with a cosmopolitan and affluent life-style
   b. cultural norms were a powerful deterrent
   c. the health hazards of tobacco became apparent

(6) Currently, in the developing world many young women have taken up smoking because _____.
   a. they practice traditional tobacco use
   b. smoking is linked with womanhood
   c. they aspire to a cosmopolitan and affluent life-style

2. passageにでてきた表現を使って次の文を英訳しなさい．
   (1) タバコの健康への害が明らかになりました．だから，あなたも喫煙をやめるべきです．　_____, so that～: _____, だから～

(2) 女性があぐらをかいて座ることは，日本では社会的に受け入れられていません．　socially unacceptable：社会的に受け入れられていない
　　　　　　　sit cross-legged：あぐらをかいて座る

(3) 女性の喫煙率の増加は女性の肺がんの死亡率の増加につながるでしょう．
　　　　　　　result in～という結果に終わる

3. 次のグラフはアメリカとスコットランドとにおける女性の肺がん死亡率と乳がん死亡率との推移を表しています．英文がグラフと一致すればTを，一致しなければFを( )に記入しなさい．

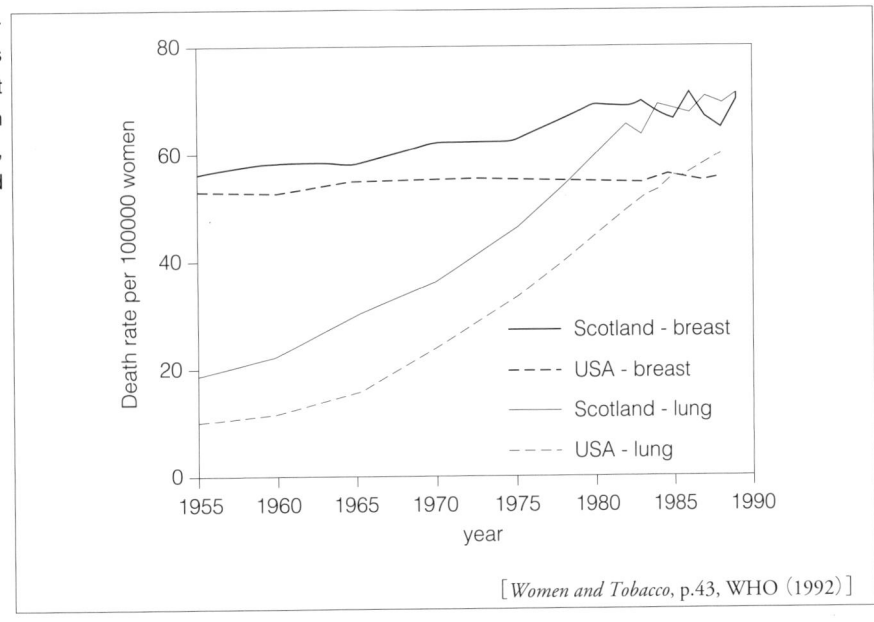

Trends in age-standardized death rates from lung and breast cancer among women aged 35–74 years, Scotland and the United States, 1955–89

[*Women and Tobacco*, p.43, WHO (1992)]

(1) In Scotland and the United State, lung cancer now accounts for more deaths among women than breast cancer. (　)

(2) The death rate from lung cancer in the United States stayed almost the same from 1955 to 1990. (　)

(3) In the United States, the death rate from lung cancer is now almost the same as that from breast cancer. (　)

(4) In Scotland and the United States, breast cancer accounted for more deaths among women than lung cancer before 1980. (　)

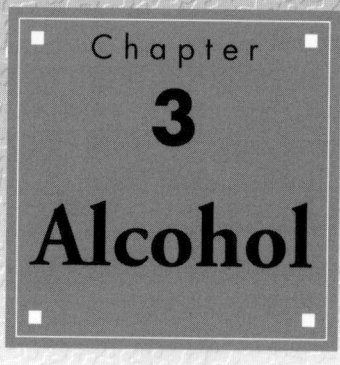

Chapter 3 Alcohol

飲酒

I. How Alcohol Acts on the Body

お酒を飲んだらどうなるの？

> Drink less, and go home by daylight.

■ Pre-reading activities

1. アメリカではblood alcohol levelすなわち，血中のアルコール含有量が飲酒運転を判断する際の基準になっています．以下はblood alcohol levelを説明する英文です．（　）の中に入る最も適切な語を枠内から選んで記入しなさい．

　　The percentage of alcohol in a person's blood is the (　　) that highway patrol officers use to determine if a driver is (　　). A blood alcohol level of ten percent or 0.10 means one part alcohol to 1,000 parts blood, which in most states is (　　) drunk, leads to a (　　) of "Driving While Intoxicated" (DWI). Even at 0.05, a drinker's driving skills aren't (　　), which has resulted in some states lowering their DWI requirement to this level. The laws vary, so make sure you know yours. At the same time, remember that individuals react (　　) to alcohol. A blood alcohol content of 0.03 isn't comfortable for everyone. It's best not to (　　) at all.　　　　　　　　　［出典B. p.51, l. 1〜9］

up to par	differently	measure	drunk	charge
drink and drive	legally			

I. How Alcohol Acts on the Body

2. ( )の中に入る最も適切な語を枠内から選んで記入しなさい。

(1) The central nervous system is located in the brain and ( ).
(2) The policemen are on the ( ) for a criminal.
(3) Drinking leads to the loss of ( ).
(4) A drinker is barely able to walk without ( ).
(5) At the highest stage of ( ), a drinker becomes unconscious.

> alert   staggering   spine   intoxication   inhibition

▪ Read the passage

次の英文は飲酒が体にどのように作用するかを説明しています。

When a person drinks one dose of alcohol, it takes about fifteen minutes for it to get to the bloodstream. This means it is carried to all parts of the body quickly—including the brain.

The brain is like the cockpit of a plane. It's the control center for our bodies, and it's very sensitive to alcohol. Doctors think alcohol depresses (stops or slows) a part of the brain that controls different parts of the body. We don't think much about being able to stand, walk, and speak with ease, but these are complex actions that are all coordinated by the central nervous system, located in the brain and spine. As the level of alcohol rises in the body, the nervous system works less and less efficiently.

After the first drink or two, (around 0.05 blood alcohol level) a drinker may only show a change in alertness, perhaps by not paying as much attention to what people around him are saying. As he has a little more, the drinker loses fine movement control—he'll spill his drink when he's trying to pour more or bump into furniture. Because drinking affects inhibitions (self-control), he might talk more or louder than usual, flirt with women he wouldn't normally flirt with, dance when he's never danced before.

When the drinker's blood alcohol content reaches a higher point (between 0.10 and 0.15), he will walk or stand unsteadily. His lack of fine movement control is even more pronounced; writing a letter, driving a car, washing dishes, having sex, or anything else involving his muscles might be hopeless. Other abilities are reduced, too: Although he can hear sounds, he might have trouble distinguishing between them and judging their direction. When he hears his wife calling, he thinks it's coming from the downstairs kitchen instead of the upstairs bedroom. Alcohol also affects the drinker's sense of time and space (five hours in a bar might seem like fifteen minutes); his vision (if he's driving, a red light won't look as red as it should); his smell and taste (he could eat a whole dinner without really paying attention to it); his emotions (he might start fights, cry over silly things, dare to do something risky, act very sexy—in other words, act on impulse or feelings rather than on thought or judgment).

As the blood alcohol content gets dangerously higher, the drinker is barely able to speak clearly or walk without staggering. His perception of pain is awry, too; if he went out in the freezing cold, he probably wouldn't feel it. He could fall and hurt himself, but he might not realize it.

At the highest stage of intoxication, a drinker becomes unconscious. When the blood alcohol percentage is more than 0.35, death is possible.

[出典 B. p.50 全文]

Notes depress：鈍らせる the central nervous system：中枢神経系 spine：背骨，ここでは脊髄（せきずい） alertness：注意深さ inhibitions：自己抑制 flirt：たわむれる pronounced：明白な impulse：衝動 stagger：よろめく perception：知覚 awry：それて，まちがって intoxication：酩酊

■ Post-reading activities

1. ＿＿＿に入る最も適切なものをa〜cから選びなさい．

   (1) When a person drinks one dose of alcohol, ＿＿＿．
      a. it takes about fifty minutes for it to get to the blood stream
      b. it is carried to all parts of the body in fifteen minutes
      c. it is carried to all parts of the body slowly

   (2) Doctors think that ＿＿＿．
      a. alcohol switches off a part of brain that controls different

parts of the body
    b. alcohol stimulates a part of brain that controls different parts of the body
    c. alcohol depresses only a part of the brain that controls speaking
(3) After the first drink or two, a drinker _____.
    a. may be cheerful
    b. may be more careful
    c. may be more careless
(4) When a drinker's blood alcohol content reaches a higher point, _____.
    a. he will walk or stand steadily
    b. his lack of fine movement control is even clearer
    c. anything involving alcohol content gets dangerously higher
(5) As the blood alcohol content gets dangerously higher, a drinker becomes _____.
    a. alert
    b. sleepy
    c. unconscious

2. passageにでてきた表現を使って次の文を英訳しなさい.
   (1) 血中のアルコールのレベルが上がるにつれて不注意になります.
       as～：～するにつれて   alert：注意深い

   (2) お酒を飲むと，しっかりと歩くのが困難になるかもしれません.
       have trouble～ing：～するのが困難である

   (3) 私は母が呼んでいるのを聞いて，階下へ降りました.
       hear ——～ing：——が～しているのを聞く

   (4) 私は車で帰るつもりだったので，お酒の代わりにジュースを飲みました.
       instead of：～の代わりに

3. 次のグラフを見てください．Aは標準的な男性が，2 ounces（約50 ml）のウィスキーを1時間ごとに4回飲んだときの血中アルコール濃度を，Bは標準的な男性が8 ounces（約227 ml）のウィスキーを一気に飲んだときの血中アルコー

ル濃度を表しています．次の英文はA，Bどちらを説明しているのでしょう．

(1) The blood alcohol concentration starts rising abruptly and reaches the highest level in the first hour; and it declines steadily.

(2) At the end of the first hour, the blood alcohol concentration has passed its peak and begun to decline, but with the next drink the concentration starts rising again; this is repeated after each drink. Only at the end of four hours is the highest blood alcohol concentration reached; and it declines steadily thereafter.

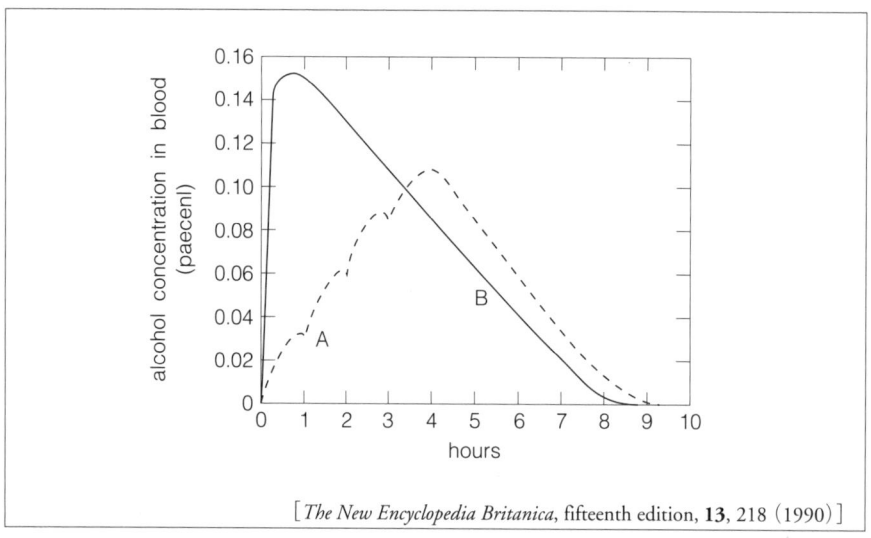

[*The New Encyclopedia Britanica*, fifteenth edition, **13**, 218 (1990)]

またこのグラフから言えることは下の(1)〜(3)のうちどれでしょう．

(1) The hazard of alcohol is higher when one drinks it quickly.

(2) The risk of alcohol is higher when one drinks for a long time.

(3) The hazard of alcohol depends on its amount.

II. Drinking in Moderation

ほどほどに飲みましょう

Is Alcoholism a Disease?

Yes. Alcoholism is a chronic, often progressive disease with symptoms that include a strong need to drink despite negative consequences, such as serious job or health problems. [NIAAA]

Notes chronic：慢性の　progressive：進行性の　symptoms：症状

■ Pre-reading activities

1. 多量のお酒を長期間飲み続けると，どのような病気になると思いますか．あてはまるものを○で囲みなさい．

   coronary heart disease   flu   cirrhosis   appendicitis
   cholera   tonsillitis   tetanus   high blood pressure
   stroke   birth defects   inflammation of the pancreas

2. (　)の中に入る最も適切なものをa〜dから選びなさい．
   (1) Infant (　) fell sharply in developed countries.
      a. dependency   b. effect   c. mortality   d. disease
   (2) Alcoholic beverages have been used to (　) the enjoyment of meals.
      a. enhance   b. decrease   c. reduce   d. do
   (3) She became (　) with their second child.
      a. dependent   b. progressive   c. pregnant   d. chronic
   (4) You have to get a (　) filled.
      a. symptom   b. syndrome   c. medication   d. prescription

Read the passage

長期に渡る飲酒は身体にさまざまな悪影響をおよぼします。したがって、飲んではいけない人もいます。

Alcohol beverages supply calories but few or no nutrients. The alcohol in these beverages has effects that are harmful when consumed in excess. These effects of alcohol may alter judgment and can lead to dependency and a great many other serious health problems. Alcohol beverages have been used to enhance the enjoyment of meals by many societies throughout human history. If adults choose to drink alcoholic beverages, they should consume them only in moderation.

Current evidence suggests that moderate drinking is associated with a lower risk for coronary heart disease in some individuals. However, higher levels of alcohol intake raise the risk for high blood pressure, stroke, heart disease, certain cancers, accidents, violence, suicides, birth defects, and overall mortality (deaths). Too much alcohol may cause cirrhosis of the liver, inflammation of the pancreas, and damage to the brain and heart. Heavy drinkers also are at risk of malnutrition because alcohol contains calories that may substitute for those in more nutritious foods.

Some people should not drink alcohol beverages at all. These include:

- Children and adolescents.
- Individuals of any age who cannot restrict their drinking to moderate levels. This is a special concern for recovering alcoholics and people whose family members have alcohol problems.
- Women who are trying to conceive or who are pregnant. Major birth defects, including fetal alcohol syndrome, have been attributed to heavy drinking by the mother while pregnant. While there is no conclusive evidence that an occasional drink is harmful to the fetus or to the pregnant woman, a safe level of alcohol intake during pregnancy has not been established.
- Individuals who plan to drive or take part in activities that require attention or skill. Most people retain some alcohol in the blood up

to 2-3 hours after a single drink.
- Individuals using prescription and over-the-counter medications. Alcohol may alter the effectiveness or toxicity of medicines. Also, some medications may increase blood alcohol levels or increase the adverse effect of alcohol on the brain. [NIAAA]

Notes　nutrient：栄養物　in excess：過度に　dependency：依存症　enhance：強める　moderation：適度　coronary heart disease：冠状動脈性心臓病　stroke：卒中　birth defects：先天性欠損　mortality：死亡率　cirrhosis：肝硬変　inflammation：炎症　pancreas：膵臓　malnutrition：栄養不良　substitute for：〜の代わりをする　alcoholic：アルコール依存症患者　conceive：妊娠する　fetal：胎児の　syndrome：症候群　prescription and over-the-counter medications：処方薬および大衆薬　toxicity：毒性　adverse effect：逆効果，悪い影響

▪ Post-reading activities

1. 本文の内容に基づいて，飲酒の利点と欠点を下の表に記入しなさい．

Advantages of drinking	Disadvantages of drinking

2. ＿＿＿に入る最も適切なものをa〜cから選びなさい．

   (1) If alcoholic beverages are consumed in excess, it ＿＿＿．
      a. will change judgment and can lead to alcoholism
      b. will supply calories with nutrients
      c. will enhance the enjoyment of meals

   (2) Current evidence suggests that ＿＿＿．
      a. even moderate drinking raises the risk of coronary heart disease
      b. moderate drinking has something to do with a lower risk of coronary heart disease in some individuals
      c. any drinking raises the risk of coronary heart disease

(3) Higher levels of alcohol intake _____.
   a. supply enough calories
   b. lower the risk of high blood pressure, stroke, heart disease, certain cancers, accident, violence, suicides, birth defects, and overall mortality
   c. may cause cirrhosis of the liver, inflammation of the pancreas and damage to the brain and heart
(4) Women who are trying to conceive or who are pregnant should not drink alcoholic beverages at all because _____.
   a. major birth defects have been due to heavy drinking by the mother while pregnant
   b. there is no conclusive evidence that an occasional drink is harmful
   c. a safe level of alcohol intake during pregnancy has been established
(5) If you have a single drink, _____.
   a. you will retain some alcohol in the blood up to 2-3 hours
   b. you will retain some alcohol in the blood up to 1-2 hours
   c. you will not retain any alcohol in the blood one hour later
(6) Individuals using prescription and over-the counter medications should not drink alcohol because _____.
   a. alcohol is harmful
   b. most people retain some alcohol in the blood up to 2-3 hours after a single drink
   c. alcohol may alter the effectiveness or toxicity of medicines

3. WHOはアルコール関係の問題を持つ人たちの初期の徴候を発見するために，The Alcohol Use Disorders Identification Test (AUDIT) というアンケートを開発しました．選んだ答えの番号の数を足してみて下さい．8点がcut-off-pointです．8点以上の人たちのうち，3分の2はこれから3年の間にアルコール関係の問題を経験するでしょう．一方，8点以下の人たちがアルコール関係の問題を経験するのは10％程度です．たった10項目からなるシンプルなものですので，身近な人たちにためしてみてください．

THE AUDIT QUESTIONNAIRE

Circle the number that comes closest to the patient's answer.

1. **How often do you have a drink containing alcohol?**
   (0) Never   (1) Monthly or less   (2) Two to four times a month
   (3) Two to three times a week   (4) Four or more times a week

2.* **How many drinks containing alcohol do you have on a typical day when you are drinking? (code number of standard drinks)**
   (0) 1 or 2   (1) 3 or 4   (2) 5 or 6   (3) 7 or 8   (4) 10 or more

3. **How often do you have six or more drinks on one occasion?**
   (0) Never   (1) Less than monthly   (2) Monthly   (3) Weekly   (4) Daily or almost daily

4. **How often during the last year have you found that you were not able to stop drinking once you had started?**
   (0) Never   (1) Less than monthly   (2) Monthly   (3) Weekly   (4) Daily or almost daily

5. **How often during the last year have you failed to do what was normally expected from you because of drinking?**
   (0) Never   (1) Less than monthly   (2) Monthly   (3) Weekly   (4) Daily or almost daily

6. **How often during the last year have you needed a first drink in the morning to get yourself going after a heavy drinking session?**
   (0) Never   (1) Less than monthly   (2) Monthly   (3) Weekly   (4) Daily or almost daily

7. **How often during the last year have you had a feeling of guilt or remorse after drinking?**
   (0) Never   (1) Less than monthly   (2) Monthly   (3) Weekly   (4) Daily or almost daily

8. **How often during the last year have you been unable to remember what happened the night before because you had been drinking?**
   (0) Never   (1) Less than monthly   (2) Monthly   (3) Weekly   (4) Daily or almost daily

9. **Have you or someone else been injured as a result of your drinking?**
   (0) No   (2) Yes, but not in the last year   (4) Yes, during the last year

10. **Has a relative or friend or a doctor or other health worker been concerned about your drinking or suggested you cut down?**
    (0) No   (2) Yes, but not in the last year   (4) Yes, during the last year

* In determining the response categories it has been assumed that one "drink" contains 10 g alcohol. In countries where the alcohol content of a standard drink differs by more than 25 % from 10 g, the response category should be modified accordingly.

Record sum of individual item scores here_____.

[Thomas F. Babor *et al.*, *AUDIT The Alcohol Use Disorders Identification Test* (Programme on Substance Abuse), p.14, WHO (1992)]

Chapter 4
HIV/AIDS

HIVとエイズ

I. What Is AIDS?

エイズってどんな病気？

FACTS

About 1.8 million adults died of AIDS in 1997 and the annual death toll is likely to rise.

■ Pre-reading activities

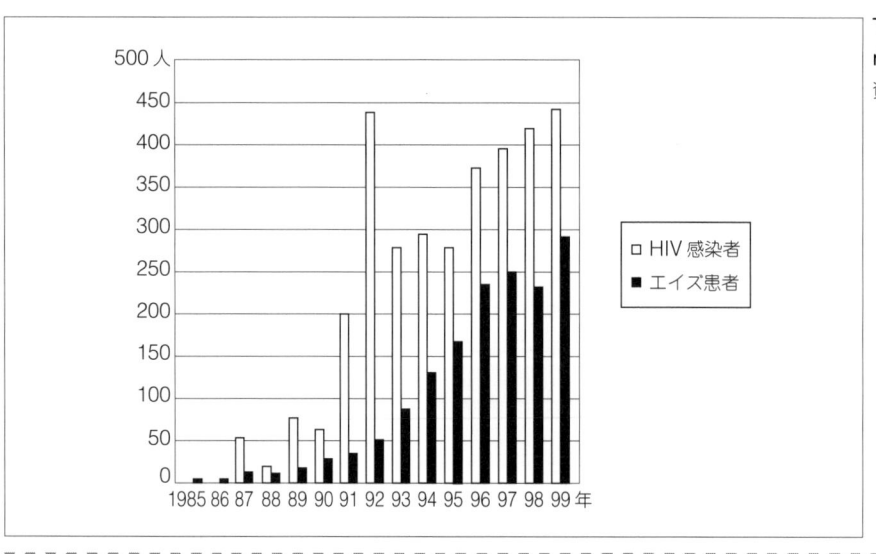

The number of HIV carriers and AIDS cases
資料：厚生省

□ HIV 感染者
■ エイズ患者

I. What Is AIDS?

1. グラフは日本のHIV感染者とエイズ患者の推移を表しています．このグラフから言えることはa～cのどれでしょう．

    a. In general, the number of those infected with HIV has increased but those with AIDS has decreased.
    b. In general, both the numbers of those infected with HIV and AIDS have been rising.
    c. In general, both the numbers of those infected with HIV and AIDS have been declining.

2. （　）の中に入る最も適切なものをa～dから選びなさい．
    (1) The HIV virus weakens the body's (　) system.
        a. nervous   b. immune   c. organ   d. muscle
    (2) The majority of (　) individuals look healthy and feel well for many years after infection.
        a. infected   b. acquired   c. contaminated
        d. screened
    (3) They may not even suspect they harbor the virus, though they can (　) to others.
        a. transfer   b. send   c. transmit   d. move
    (4) <u>Antiretroviral</u> (　) is not available to most people in the developing world.
        a. disease   b. method   c. infection   d. therapy

Notes　antiretroviral：抗レトロウイルスの

▪Read the passage

以下の英文はUNAIDS（国連合同エイズ計画）がエイズについて説明したものです．エイズとはどういう病気なのか，正確な知識をもってください．

AIDS stands for "<u>acquired immunodeficiency syndrome</u>"—a syndrome being a cluster of <u>medical conditions</u>. It is caused by the human <u>immunodeficiency virus</u> (HIV), which weakens the body's immune system.

HIV spreads through unprotected sex (intercourse without a condom), transfusions of unscreened blood, <u>contaminated</u> needles (most frequently for injecting drug use), and from an infected woman to her child during pregnancy, childbirth or breast-feeding.

HIV is a slow-acting virus. The majority of infected individuals look healthy and feel well for many years after infection; they may not even suspect they harbor the virus, though they can transmit it to others. Conservative UNAIDS estimates are that 90 % of all HIV-infected people worldwide do not know they have the virus. A laboratory blood or saliva test is the only certain way to determine whether an individual is HIV-positive.

Once they have an established HIV infection, individuals are infected for life and will probably succumb to serious opportunistic infections caused by the weakening of their immune system. Treatment with antiretroviral drugs can slow the progression of HIV infection but these expensive medications are not available to most people in the developing world, who often lack access even to drugs that combat opportunistic infections. In individuals who do not get antiretroviral therapy, the time between infection with HIV and the development of the serious illnesses that define AIDS is around eight years, and most patients do not survive much more than two years after the onset of AIDS.

[出典D. p.10 全文]

Notes　acquired immunodeficiency syndrome：後天性免疫不全症候群　medical conditions：病状　immunodeficiency virus：免疫不全ウイルス　contaminate：汚染する　slow-acting：遅延性の　harbor：宿す　conservative：控えめな　UNAIDS：The Joint United Nations Programme on HIV/AIDS, 国連合同エイズ計画（programmeは英式つづり．米式はprogram）　saliva：だ液　HIV-positive：HIV検査が陽性の　succumb to：屈する　opportunistic infections：日和見感染症（宿主の抵抗力が弱まった時だけ発症する）　antiretroviral drug：抗レトロウイルス薬　medication：医薬

■ Post-reading activities

1. 次の質問に英語で答えなさい．

　(1) What is AIDS?

　(2) How is HIV transmitted?

(3) Do all HIV-infected people worldwide know they have the virus? Why?

(4) How are antiretroviral drugs helpful for HIV-infected people?

(5) How long does it take for an HIV-infected person to develop serious illnesses that define AIDS without antiretroviral drugs?

(6) How long do most AIDS patients survive after the onset of AIDS?

2. passageにでてきた表現を使って次の文を英訳しなさい．
   (1) WHOはWorld Health Organizationの略です．
        stand for：〜の略である，〜を表す

   (2) いったん，医師の免許をとれば，一生医者をすることができます．
        once〜：いったん〜をすれば

   (3) この図書館は一般の人は利用できません．
        available to〜：〜には利用できる

3. 次の行為のうち，HIVが感染する可能性のあるものはどれでしょう．
- hugging a person
- sitting on a toilet seat
- being stung by mosquitoes
- unprotected sexual intercourse
- breast-feeding by an infected woman
- an infected woman to her child during pregnancy
- donating blood
- transfusions of unscreened blood
- contaminated needles (most frequently for injecting drug use)

II. The Global Plague of AIDS

エイズの世界的な広がり

FACTS

A large proportion of the deaths occurring between the ages of 15 and 59 years in low and middle income countries can be attributed to HIV and tuberculosis.

■ Pre-reading activities

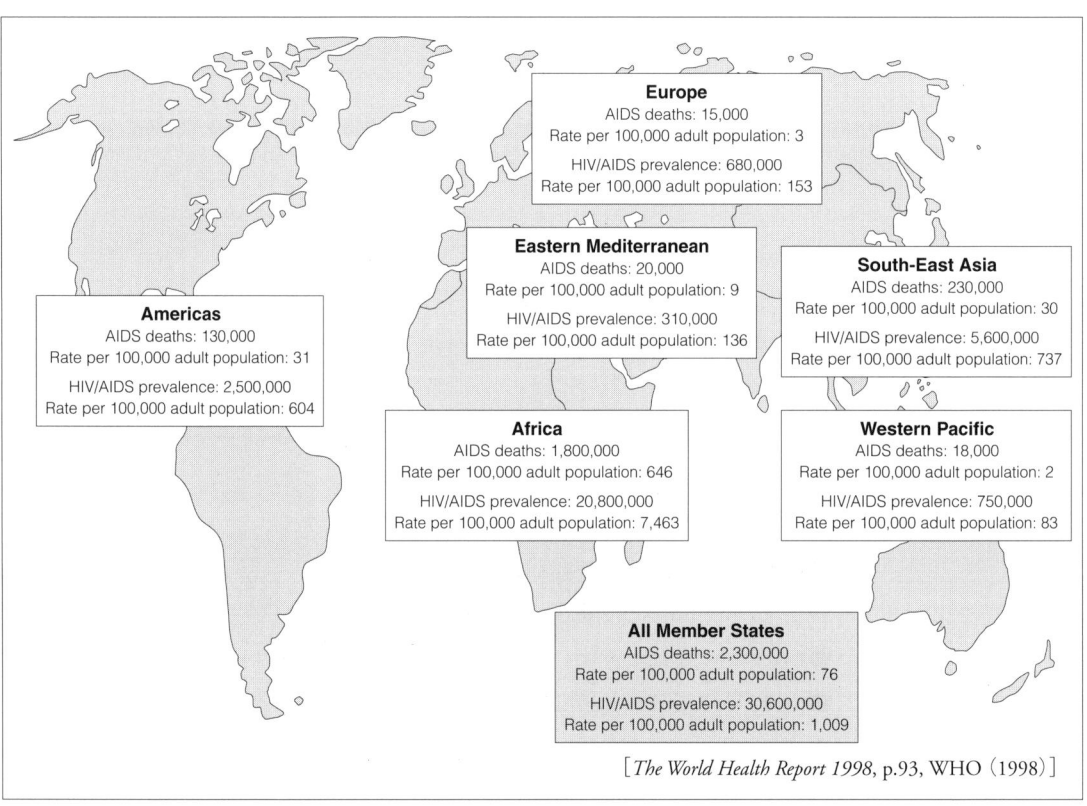

Europe
AIDS deaths: 15,000
Rate per 100,000 adult population: 3

HIV/AIDS prevalence: 680,000
Rate per 100,000 adult population: 153

Eastern Mediterranean
AIDS deaths: 20,000
Rate per 100,000 adult population: 9

HIV/AIDS prevalence: 310,000
Rate per 100,000 adult population: 136

South-East Asia
AIDS deaths: 230,000
Rate per 100,000 adult population: 30

HIV/AIDS prevalence: 5,600,000
Rate per 100,000 adult population: 737

Americas
AIDS deaths: 130,000
Rate per 100,000 adult population: 31

HIV/AIDS prevalence: 2,500,000
Rate per 100,000 adult population: 604

Africa
AIDS deaths: 1,800,000
Rate per 100,000 adult population: 646

HIV/AIDS prevalence: 20,800,000
Rate per 100,000 adult population: 7,463

Western Pacific
AIDS deaths: 18,000
Rate per 100,000 adult population: 2

HIV/AIDS prevalence: 750,000
Rate per 100,000 adult population: 83

All Member States
AIDS deaths: 2,300,000
Rate per 100,000 adult population: 76

HIV/AIDS prevalence: 30,600,000
Rate per 100,000 adult population: 1,009

[*The World Health Report 1998*, p.93, WHO (1998)]

AIDS deaths and HIV/AIDS prevalence among adults aged 15-49, by WHO region, 1997 estimates

1. 図と一致する英文にはTを，一致しない英文にはFを（　）に記入しなさい．

   (1) Europe has the smallest rate of HIV-infected people per 100,000 adult population. (　)
   (2) Africa has the largest number of AIDS deaths. (　)
   (3) More than 30 million people are infected with HIV all over the world. (　)
   (4) The number of people infected with HIV in Americas is about half of that in South-East Asia, and the rate per 100,000 adult population is also about half. (　)
   (5) More people are infected with HIV in Europe than in Americas. (　)

2. (　)に入る最も適切なものをa〜dから選びなさい．

   (1) The United Nations (　) that 90 percent of them are unaware of their infection.
       a. guesses   b. counts   c. estimates   d. establishes
   (2) New AIDS (　) are emerging with exponential speed in many regions.
       a. epidemics   b. fashions   c. vogues   d. heritages
   (3) In some countries in East and southern Africa, a quarter of the adult population is (　) with AIDS.
       a. moved   b. transmitted   c. contaminated   d. infected
   (4) It would cost a lot of money to do an adequate job of AIDS (　).
       a. prevention   b. privilege   c. prescription   d. medicine

▪▪ Read the passage

　エイズの蔓延は社会的，経済的な要素と深くかかわっています．特に，貧困がエイズの予防と治療を妨げています．

　By the end of 1999, more than 33 million people worldwide were living with H.I.V., the virus that causes AIDS, though the United Nations <u>estimates</u> that 90 percent of them are unaware of their infection. More than 16 million have died. Sub-Saharan Africa remains the worst off, with more than 23 million infected and 14 million dead. But new AIDS epidemics are emerging with exponential speed in Eastern and Central Europe, in India and China, and throughout Southeast Asia, Latin America and the Caribbean.

For many of these regions, AIDS is more than just a humanitarian problem, it is decimating not the elderly and infirm, but the most vibrant and economically productive sector of the population. In some countries in East and southern Africa, a quarter of the adult population is infected, with infection rates highest among skilled and semi-skilled workers, including doctors and nurses, teachers, engineers and civil servants.

In much of the developing world, treatment for the disease is negligible. Fewer than 10 percent of infected Africans are getting so much as an aspirin tablet to stem the ravages of tuberculosis, pneumonia and brain infections that accompany AIDS. There is still no cure for AIDS and no vaccine. The powerful drug cocktails that are prolonging lives among H.I.V. positive people in developed countries can cost as much as $15,000 a year for a single patient. Drug companies could help by reducing prices for the poorest regions, but even prices reduced by 90 percent would be unaffordable for Africans whose annual income is counted in the hundreds of dollars.

The highest priority now is to arrest the alarming spread of the disease. The U.N. estimates it would cost between $2 billion and $3 billion a year to do an adequate job of prevention in developing countries. The U.N. and international lending agencies have already committed substantial sums to AIDS prevention, but current efforts are reaching only 10 to 20 percent of vulnerable populations. The United States has nearly doubled its own contribution to global AIDS prevention efforts, from $125 million per year over the last several years to $235 million this year. There is bipartisan support in Congress for bills that would authorize $2 billion more over the next five years.

The increases are laudable, but they will not be sufficient. Currently, some 95 percent of all the AIDS prevention money is being spent in the industrialized countries, while 95 percent of those infected live in the developing countries.

[出典 E. L 20～R 21]

Notes estimate：見積もる infection：感染 epidemic：流行 emerge：現れる exponential speed：ものすごいスピード(exponentialは指数関数のこと) humanitarian：人道的な decimate：～の多くを殺す infirm：虚弱な vibrant：活力のある negligible：無いに等しい stem：阻止する ravages：荒廃 tuberculosis：結核 pneumonia：肺炎 accompany：伴う unaffordable：買うことができない arrest：阻止する prevention：予防 international lending agencies：国際的な融資機関 commit：ゆだねる substantial：相当な vulnerable：感染しやすい bipartisan：超党派の laudable：賞賛すべき

■ Post-reading activities

1. ＿＿に入る最も適切なものをa～cから選びなさい.

   (1) By the end of 1999, more than 33 million people worldwide were living with H.I.V., though ＿＿.
       a. the United Nations estimates that 90 percent of them are aware of their infection
       b. the United Nations estimates that 90 percent of them have not noticed their infection
       c. the United Nations estimates that 90 percent of them are weakened by their infection

   (2) New AIDS epidemics ＿＿.
       a. have not emerged throughout the world
       b. are surging at a terrible speed in many regions
       c. are emerging especially in China

   (3) In many regions, AIDS is more than just a humanitarian problem because ＿＿.
       a. treatment for the disease requires a lot of money
       b. it is killing the elderly and infirm
       c. it is killing the most economically productive sector of the population

   (4) In much of the developing world, ＿＿.
       a. the medicines for prolonging lives among H.I.V. positive people are unaffordable

b. many H.I.V. positive people can afford to buy the powerful drug cocktails

c. about 90 percent of infected people are not getting so much as an aspirin tablet to stem the ravages of tuberculosis, pneumonia and brain infections that accompany AIDS

(5) The U.N. and international lending agencies have already committed substantial sum to AIDS prevention but ＿＿＿.

a. only 10 to 20 percent of the money is reaching vulnerable populations

b. that sum of money is enough for only 10 to 20 percent of susceptible people

c. it is negligible compared to the United States efforts for global AIDS prevention

(6) Some 95 percent of those infected live in the developing countries, ＿＿＿.

a. and the AIDS prevention money is being spent according to the number of the patients

b. and some 95 percent of all the AIDS prevention money is being spent in the industrialized countries

c. and some 95 percent of all the AIDS prevention money is being spent in the developing countries

2. passageにでてきた表現を使って次の文を英訳しなさい．

（1）政府はその地震による被害は30億円を超えると見積もっています．
　　　estimate：見積もる

（2）エイズ予防の資金は発展途上国ではなく，先進国でより多く使われています．　　not～but ―：～ではなく―

（3）エイズのための薬は高いので，発展途上国の人々は買うことができません．
　　　unaffordable：買うことができない

3. 健康に対する政策を立案するには，ある集団の健康状態を測定する必要があります．そのためにWorld BankとWorld Health Organization (WHO) により開発されたのがDALYです．DALYとはDisability-Adjusted Life Years－「障害調整生存年数」のことで，早死にや障害や病気により失われた年数を表しています．DALYはある集団の健康にとって，早死にや障害や病気がどのくらいの比重を占めるのかを示します．

下のグラフは，低所得，中所得の国々におけるDALYの内訳を表しています．HIV/AIDSはおとなのDALYの何パーセントを占めていますか．

DALYs attributable to conditions in the unfinished agenda in low and middle income countries, estimates for 1998

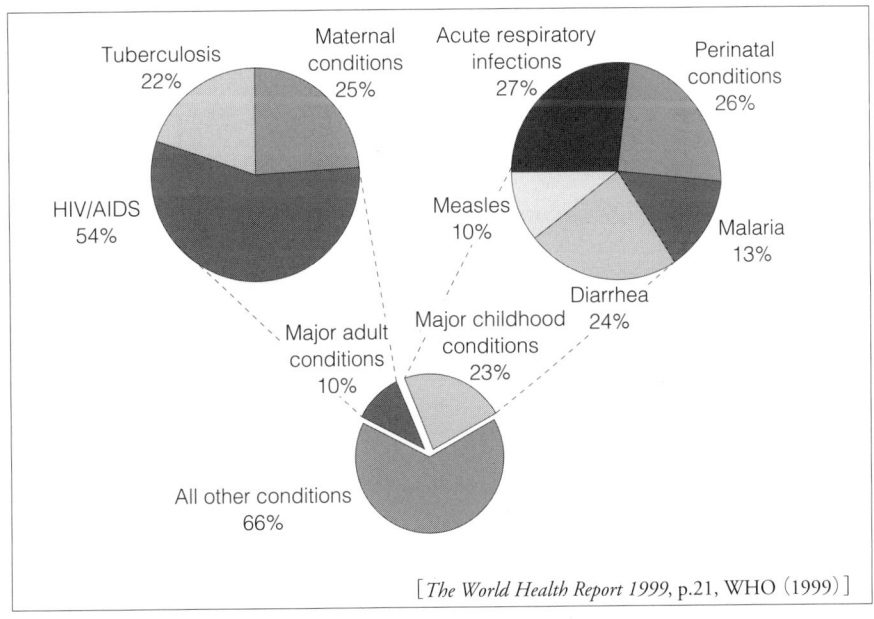

Tuberculosis 22%
Maternal conditions 25%
Acute respiratory infections 27%
Perinatal conditions 26%
HIV/AIDS 54%
Measles 10%
Malaria 13%
Diarrhea 24%
Major adult conditions 10%
Major childhood conditions 23%
All other conditions 66%

[*The World Health Report 1999*, p.21, WHO (1999)]

Chapter 5 Nutrition

栄養

I. Diet Is Important to Health

食事は健康にとってたいせつなもの

> Food is required as a fuel for the maintenance of energy-requiring processes that sustain life.

Notes　maintenance：維持　sustain：支える

■ Pre-reading activities

1. 下の図は消化器官を表しています．各々の器官名を日本語で言いなさい．

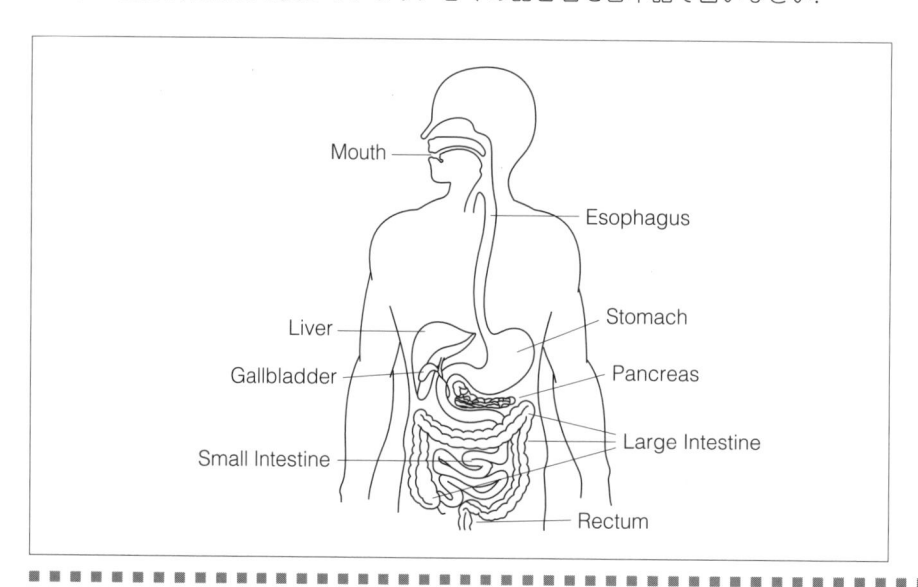

- Mouth
- Esophagus
- Liver
- Stomach
- Gallbladder
- Pancreas
- Small Intestine
- Large Intestine
- Rectum

2. （　）の中に入る最も適切なものをa～dから選びなさい．

(1) He did a little exercise to aid his (　).
 a. suggestion　　b. nutrition　　c. digestion
 d. ingestion

(2) The bumper (　) most of the shock of impact.
 a. absolute　　b. absorbed　　c. observed　　d. inhaled

(3) The rise in stock prices (　) the economy of the country.
 a. boosted　　b. hightened　　c. lowered　　d. made

(4) Some people died of (　) during the World War II.
 a. starvation　　b. fracture　　c. theft　　d. insomnia

■ Read the passage

私たちの体にとって食べ物はどのような働きをしているのでしょう．

What really happens when you eat?

After that hot dog disappeared into your mouth, it made its way down the esophagus, through the stomach and into the small intestine, where the major part of digestion takes place: Food is broken down into nutrients small enough to be absorbed into the bloodstream. The bloodstream carries the nutrients to all parts of the body, and that's where you get the energy to do the things you do every day. Nutrition not only boosts the muscles you use, it also provides energy to keep up the things you don't think about: The building and repairing of cells and the movement of blood through your body.

What really happens when you don't eat?

In the time between the bowl of cereal you ate this morning to the hot dog you ate during the third quarter, your body was still functioning. Humans aren't like cars; we can keep going for a while, even when no fuel is provided. However, you weren't operating at peak energy because without food, your blood sugar level dropped. The result: You felt tired and irritable. Unfed, your body began to reach out for the next best thing—stored fat and the protein in your muscles and organs. This weakens you and could eventually make you sick. Some recent research also shows that you might be increasing your chance of gaining weight. Your body thinks it's starving when you don't eat, so it slows down and saves all the food you ate yesterday and before. By the time you do eat, it's stockpiled for the next bout of starvation.

[出典 F. p.14, *l*. 1～8, p.15, *l*. 1～10]

Notes
esophagus：食道　digestion：消化　nutrients：栄養素　keep up：続ける　blood sugar level：血糖値　irritable：いらいらした　stockpile：備蓄する　bout：期間　starvation：飢え

■ Post-reading activities

1. 以下の質問に対して最も適切な答えを選びなさい．

    (1) Where does the major part of digestion take place?
        a. esophagus
        b. stomach
        c. small intestines

    (2) What carries the nutrients to all parts of the body?
        a. bloodstream
        b. lymph
        c. small intestines

    (3) Where do you get the energy to do the things you do every day?
        a. muscle
        b. small intestines
        c. all parts of the body

    (4) How do we feel when our blood sugar level has dropped?
        a. We feel tired and irritable.
        b. We feel depressed.
        c. We feel hungry.

    (5) What happens when you do not eat for a long time?
        a. We might be decreasing our chance of gaining weight.
        b. Our body starts to store fat and protein in our muscles and organs.
        c. Our blood sugar level rises.

I. Diet Is Important to Health

2. 以下の質問の答えを，続く英文からみつけなさい．

(1) What kind of products should be avoided in order to decrease the risk of cancer?

(2) What kind of food should be eaten in order to decrease the risk of cancer?

(3) What helps prevent cancer?

(4) What have been shown to cause cancer in animals?

(5) What is the ticket to feeling good and staying healthy?

　Here's how scientists see the food-cancer connection: When the diet is high in fat and cholesterol, bacteria inside of us break it down into cancer-causing substances. In our world, it's hard to avoid all fatty and cholesterol-heavy foods, so doctors advise us to cut down as much as possible on fat and cholesterol and to load up on fiber-rich foods. Fiber works against cancer because it comes from plants, and some plant parts can't be digested. Those parts bulk up your waste and speed it out of the body. With it, the waste takes along those cancerous substances that might have stuck to the colon (the path out of the body). Fiber helps get rid of many of these cancerous substances because it moves them out quicker than usual.

　We also know that vitamins A and C help prevent cancer. At the same time, other substances, such as food preservatives, have been shown to cause cancer in animals. Do they affect humans? Some do, some we're not sure of. Research to answer these and other questions about cancer is ongoing, which is why it's important to remember that no one vitamin or nutrient has been proven to absolutely prevent cancer. While we're still learning, it doesn't hurt to say over and over again: A high-fiber, low-fat diet is the ticket to feeling good and staying healthy.

[出典 F. p.15, R8〜23, p.16, L1〜13]

5：Nutrition

3. passageにでてきた表現を使って次の文を英訳しなさい．
（1）栄養失調は栄養を十分にとらなかったときにおこります．
mal-nutrition：栄養失調　　take place：おこる

（2）塩分の取りすぎは血圧を押し上げます．　　boost：押し上げる

（3）偏った食事をしていると結局は病気になります．
imbalanced diet：偏った食事　　eventually：結局は

II. Food Guide Pyramid

フードガイドピラミッド

Better Nutrition for Mature Adults

- Drink 6-8 glasses of water every day.
- Eat calcium rich foods, such as milk cheese, yogurt, fish with bones, and some dark green vegetables, like broccoli. Calcium is important for strong bones.
- Get plenty of Vitamin A and Vitamin C by eating fresh fruits and vegetables, such as carrots and oranges. Vitamin A is good for your eyes and skin. Vitamin C keeps gums healthy and prevents against infection.
- Eat foods high in iron, which helps the body use energy. Iron is abundant in red meat, poultry, fish, and dried beans.
- Include meats, seafood, and poultry in your diet to protect against <u>Zinc</u> deficiency. Zinc helps wounds heal faster.
- Practice regular physical activity. Outdoor activity is best, because your body can make vitamin D with the help of the sun.

[The USDA Food and Consumer Service]

Notes　zinc：亜鉛

Pre-reading activities

1. 以下は5大栄養素です．対応する英語を右から選びなさい．

    糖質（　　　　　）　　　　vitamin
    タンパク質（　　　　　）　　fat
    脂質（　　　　　）　　　　carbohydrate
    ビタミン（　　　　　）　　mineral
    ミネラル（　　　　　）　　protein

2. 次の食品の名前を英語で言ってみましょう．それぞれ，どの栄養素を最も多く含んでいますか．

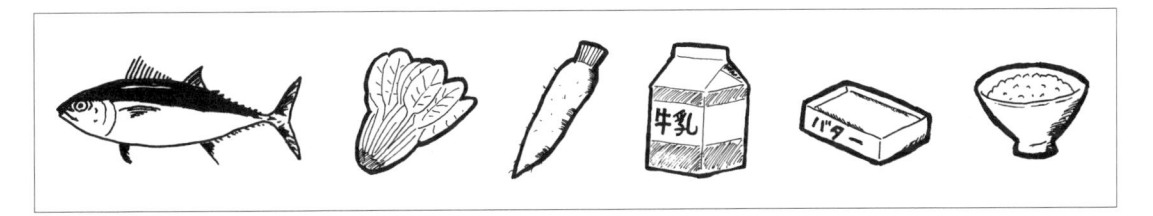

Read the passage

　健康に良い食生活を送るために，アメリカにはFood Guide Pyramidというものがあります．Food Guide Pyramidとはどういうもので，どのようにして使うのでしょう．

　Healthful diets contain the amounts of essential nutrients and calories needed to prevent nutritional <u>deficiencies</u> and <u>excesses</u>. Healthful diets also provide the right balance of carbohydrate, fat, and protein to reduce risks for chronic diseases, and are a part of a full and productive lifestyle. Such diets are obtained from a variety of foods that are available, <u>affordable</u>, and enjoyable.

　To obtain the nutrients and other substances needed for good health, vary the foods you eat. Foods contain combinations of nutrients and other healthful substances. No single food can supply all nutrients in the amounts you need. For example, oranges provide vitamin C but no vitamin B12; cheese provides vitamin B12 but no vitamin C. To make sure you get all of the nutrients and other substances needed for health, choose the recommended number of daily servings from each of the five major food groups displayed in the Food Guide Pyramid.

Use foods from the base of the Food Guide Pyramid as the foundation of your meals. However, people often choose higher or lower amounts from some food groups than suggested in the Food Guide Pyramid. The Pyramid shows that foods from the grain products group, along with vegetables and fruits, are the basis of healthful diets. Enjoy meals that have rice, pasta, potatoes, or bread at the center of the plate, accompanied by other vegetables and fruits, and lean and low-fat foods from the other groups. Limit fats and sugars added in food preparation and at the table. Compare the recommended number of servings with what you usually eat.

Choose different foods within each food group. You can achieve a healthful, nutritious eating pattern with many combinations of foods from the five major food groups. Choosing a variety of foods within and across food groups improves dietary patterns because foods within the same group have different combinations of nutrients and other beneficial substances. For example, some vegetables and fruits are good sources of vitamin C or vitamin A, while others are high in folate; still others are good sources of calcium or iron. Choosing a variety of foods

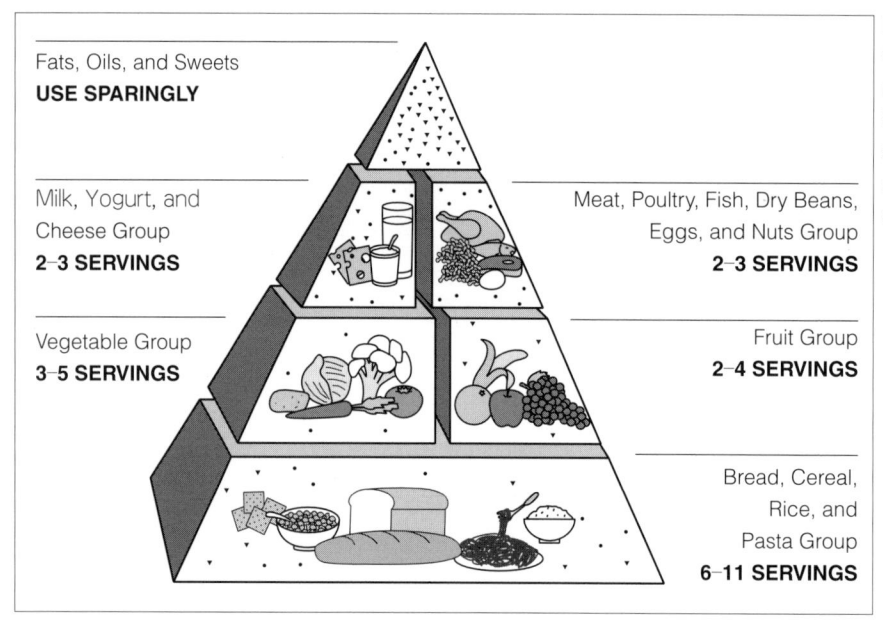

Food guide pyramid
●: Fat (naturally occurring and added), ▼: Sugars (added). These symbols show fat and added sugars in foods source: USDA

Fats, Oils, and Sweets
USE SPARINGLY

Milk, Yogurt, and Cheese Group
2–3 SERVINGS

Meat, Poultry, Fish, Dry Beans, Eggs, and Nuts Group
2–3 SERVINGS

Vegetable Group
3–5 SERVINGS

Fruit Group
2–4 SERVINGS

Bread, Cereal, Rice, and Pasta Group
6–11 SERVINGS

within each group also helps to make your meals more interesting from day to day. 　　　　　　　　　　　　　　　　　　　　　［出典 URL①，URL②］

Notes　deficiencies：不足　excesses：過剰　affordable：手に入る　folate：葉酸

▪▪ Post-reading activities

1. 次の質問に対して最も適切な答えを選びなさい．

    (1) What are healthful diets?
        a. Healthful diets are delicious when eating.
        b. Healthful diets contain the amounts of essential nutrients and calories needed to prevent nutritional deficiencies and excesses.
        c. Healthful diets contain less fat.

    (2) What is the Food Guide Pyramid?
        a. The Food Guide Pyramid is a general guide that lets you choose a healthy diet that is right for you.
        b. The Food Guide Pyramid is a chart to classify foods.
        c. The Food Guide Pyramid is a general guide that lets you know the correct calories of foods.

    (3) What should we do in order to obtain the nutrients and other substances needed for good health?
        a. We should eat much protein.
        b. We should eat what we like.
        c. We should vary the foods we eat.

    (4) What should we use as the foundation of our meals?
        a. We should use foods from the base of the Food Guide Pyramid as the foundation of our meals.
        b. We should use foods containing much protein.
        c. We should use foods from the top of the Food Guide Pyramid as the foundation of our meals.

    (5) Why should we choose a variety of foods within and across food groups in the Food Guide Pyramid?
        a. Because a single food can provide a variety of nutrients.
        b. Because foods within the same group have the same combi-

nation of nutrients and other beneficial substances.
   c. Because foods within the same group have different combination of nutrients and other beneficial substances.

2. passageにでてきた表現を使って次の文を英訳しなさい．
   （1）野菜や果物はビタミンCやビタミンAを供給するが，魚や肉はタンパク質を供給する．　　provide：供給する

   （2）あらゆる栄養素を確実にとるためには，1日30種類の食品をとれば良いといわれている．　　to make sure：〜を確実にするために

   （3）日本の平均的な食事と比べると，アメリカの平均的な食事は脂肪が多い．
         compared with：〜と比べると

3. あなたが昨日食べたものとFood Guide Pyramidが勧める食事とを比べなさい．

4. 以下の英文は栄養学的にみて，正しいでしょうか．もしまちがっているのならばどこがまちがっているのかを指摘しなさい．
   （1）Monica knows that whole-wheat pancakes are good for her, so she made some for breakfast. With butter and syrup, she couldn't even tell the difference in the taste from regular pancakes.
   （2）Boiled eggs are not cooked with oil like fried ones are, so Allen has two every morning.
   （3）Thelma has been drinking sodas that have added fruit juices ever since they first came out; she figures she'll get more vitamins from them.
   （4）Phil is trying to lose weight, so he eats frozen yogurt with fruit every day at lunch.
   （5）When Pat found out that spaghetti was healthy, she was thrilled. She eats it as often as she can, trying out different toppings: tomato sauces; butter and garlic; ground beef; and creamy cheese sauce.　　　　　　　　　　　　　［出典 F. p.79, l. 1〜12］

Chapter 6
Obesity

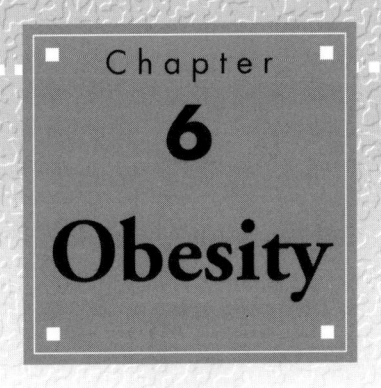

肥満

I. Why Do People Get Fat?

肥満とは？

FACTS

An obese Stone Age statue has been <u>unearthed</u>. Similar evidence of <u>obesity</u> is found in Egyptian <u>mummies</u> and in Greek <u>sculpture</u>. People in a society become obese as soon as enough food and leisure are available to cause an imbalance between energy <u>intake</u> and energy <u>expenditure</u>.

Notes unearth：出土する obesity：肥満 mummies：ミイラ sculpture：彫像 intake：摂取 expenditure：支出

■ Pre-reading activities

Checking your body shape

1. 次のグラフを見て，あなた自身と４人の若者の体型判定をしなさい．

obese	ふとりすぎ―肥満
overweight	ふとりぎみ
normal	ふつう
underweight	やせぎみ
thin	やせすぎ―やせ

6 : Obesity

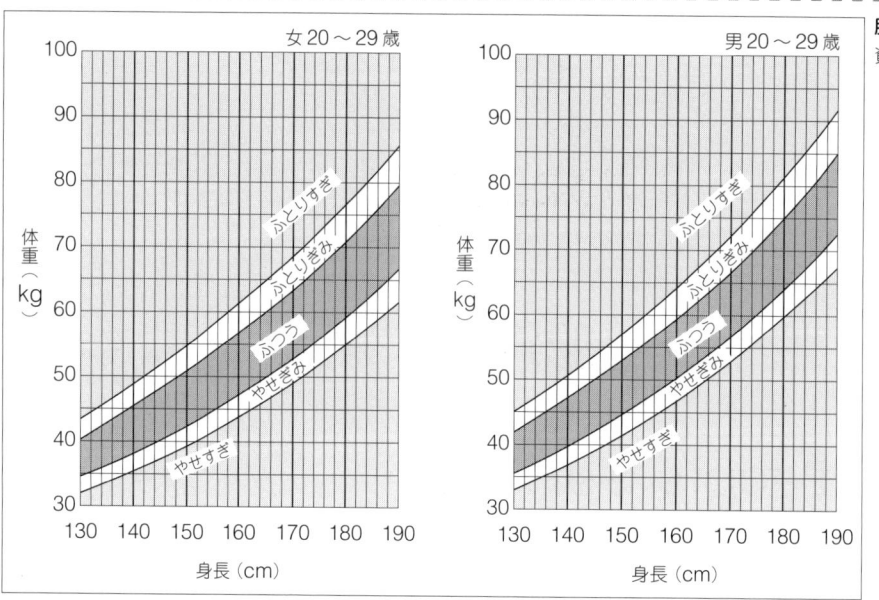

肥満とやせの判定グラフ
資料：厚生省(1986)

	Age	Weight (kg)	Height (cm)	Status
Yukiko	21	56	155	
Mari	20	65	160	
Koichi	20	55	174	
Kazuo	26	61	168	
You				

2. 肥満になるのは，自分のからだが必要とする以上のカロリー（エネルギー）をとった結果です．次の運動をカロリー消費の大きいものから，順位を付けなさい．

walking (　　)　　cross-country skiing (　　)　　sleeping (　　)
bicycling (　　)　　roller skating (　　)　　studying (　　)

■ Read the passage

Why do people get fat?

　　Calories, as you know, are the energy food <u>releases</u> into your body. You will burn some calories by simply reading a book or watching television; it takes calories for all your body functions (heart, digestion, breathing) to function smoothly. You will burn more calories by walking to school or mopping the floor, because you are using muscles. And you will burn even more calories by swimming or playing tennis,

Activity	Calories Burned Per Minute
Sleeping	1
Studying	2.2
Piano playing	3.2
Walking	5.4
Bicycling	6.7
Roller skating (fast)	11.2
Rope skipping	13.3
Cross-country skiing	16.7

because you are breathing harder, working your heart harder, and moving your muscles more.

In a nutshell, the reason people get fat is that they eat more calories than their bodies burn. One solution, of course, is to cut back on calories. Another is to increase exercise. The best answer of all: Cut calories and increase your exercise regimen.

Even if you are not on a weight-loss plan, exercise helps your body burn calories efficiently. It is a relationship we can not ignore. This chart will give you some idea of how calories are used. ［出典 F. p.102, l. 2〜14］

Young Japanese men losing war on weight

As the battle of the bulge heats up, Japan's young men find themselves increasingly under attack from obesity.

The total number of overweight people 15 years old or older, regardless of gender, reached 23 million in 1998, while the number of obese males between the ages of 15 and 39 has nearly doubled over a 19-year period, according to the Ministry of Health and Welfare.

A national survey of dietary habits conducted by the ministry in 1998 found the ratio of underweight women between 15 and 29 years old had increased since the previous survey in 1979, apparently due to their obsession with slimness.

Of the 23 million officially declared obese, 13 million are male and 10 million are female, meaning that one in four men is overweight and slightly fewer than one in five women is too heavy.

Comparing the results with those of the 1979 survey, the ratio of overweight men in the 15 to 19 age bracket increased from 6 to 11.4 percent in 1998. The figure for those in their 20s grew from 9.2 percent to 19 percent, and that of men in their 30s expanded from 16.3 percent to 30.6 percent.

In the case of women, however, the percentage of underweight <u>individuals</u> between 15 and 19 years of age increased from the previous survey's 13.5 percent to 20.4 percent. As for women in their 20s, the ratio jumped from 14.4 percent to 20.3 percent.

［出典G. 全文］

Notes　　release：放出する　in a nutshell：簡単にまとめると　cut back on：減らす　exercise regimen：実行予定の運動量　efficiently：効率よく　the battle of the bulge：ぜい肉とのたたかい（"the Battle of the Bulge" は第二次世界大戦中, 深く侵攻した独軍による猛反攻の戦闘を指す）　Ministry of Health and Welfare：厚生省　obsession：こだわり　individuals：人々

■ Post-reading activities

1. ＿＿＿＿に入る最も適切なものをa～cから選びなさい.

　(1) Calories are ＿＿＿ released into your body.
　　a. nutrients
　　b. fever
　　c. energy

　(2) You'll burn more calories by walking to school than by ＿＿＿ .
　　a. rope skipping
　　b. simply watching television
　　c. riding to school on a bicycle.

　(3) The total number of overweight people 15 years old or older reached 23 million in ＿＿＿ .
　　a. 1975
　　b. 1984
　　c. 1998

　(4) The ratio of underweight women between 14 and 29 years old increased since the previous survey in 1979, apparently due to ＿＿＿ .
　　a. a lack of an adequate food supply.

b. their ignorance of nutritional needs.

c. their obsession with slimness.

(5) The ratio of _____ increased from 6 in 1979 to 11.4 percent in 1998.

a. overweight males between 15 and 19

b. underweight females in the 15 to 19 age bracket

c. overweight males between the ages of 15 and 39

(6) The ratio of underweight women in their 20s has jumped from 14.4 to 20.3 percent _____ .

a. in 1998

b. over a 19-year period

c. over 15 years.

2. 英文では，同じ単語や語句を，あまり間隔をおかない箇所でくりかえして使うのは，よい英作文ではないとされます．次の単語は，本文中ではどのような同じ意味の別の単語に置き換えられているでしょうか．

(1) obesity (　　　　)　　(2) men (　　　　)

(3) women (　　　　)　　(4) increase (　　　　)

(5) underweight (　　　　)　　(6) expand (　　　　)

(7) individuals (　　　　)

3. passageにでてきた表現を使って次の文を英訳しなさい．

(1) 50〜59歳までの，やせている人の数は6.0％から2.8％に減少した．
　　　underweight people：やせている人

(2) 厚生省がおこなった国民栄養調査によれば，20，30歳代の肥満者が著しく増加した．
　　　national survey of dietary habits：国民栄養調査
　　　increased remarkably：著しく増加した

(3) 15〜19歳の日本女性の5人に1人はやせすぎであるが，一方，ふとりすぎは20人に1人よりわずかに多いのみである．
　　　while〜：一方〜である

6 : Obesity

II. Indices of Overweight

肥満をはかる指数

FACTS

Growth in the number of severely overweight adults is expected to be double that of underweight adults during 1995-2050.

Pre-reading activities

1. 次のグラフは世界のいくつかの国々の肥満とやせの割合（％）を表しています．下の質問に英語で答えなさい．

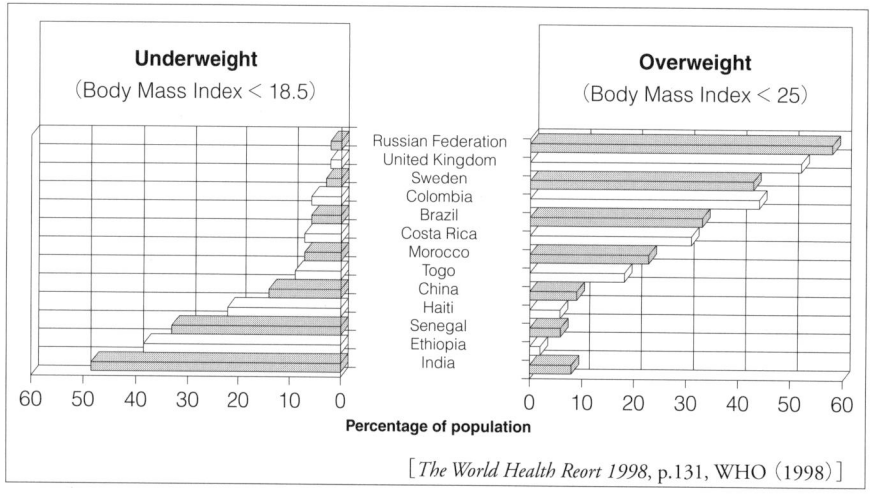

Underweight (Body Mass Index < 18.5)

Overweight (Body Mass Index < 25)

Russian Federation, United Kingdom, Sweden, Colombia, Brazil, Costa Rica, Morocco, Togo, China, Haiti, Senegal, Ethiopia, India

Percentage of population underweight and overweight, selected countries, around 1993

[*The World Health Reort 1998*, p.131, WHO (1998)]

(1) How many countries have more overweight people in their populations than underweight people?

(2) What country has the greatest percentage of underweight people? And what country has the greatest percentage of overweight people?

(3) In how many countries is the percentage of the overweight population greater than 25%?

■ Read the passage

肥満も度が過ぎればひとつの立派な病気と見なされます．その境界はどこにあるのでしょうか．肥満をはかる尺度としてBMIというものがあります．

How is obesity to be measured?

The BMI is obtained by dividing the weight in kilograms by height measured in meters, squared (W/H^2). Identical standard values can be used for all adult patients, both men and women. The lowest morbidity and mortality, for both sexes occur in persons with a BMI of 22-25 kg/m^2.

Obesity (BMI > 30) is a disease that is largely preventable through changes in lifestyle. Overweight (BMI > 25) is a major determinant of many NCDs including NIDDM, CHD and stroke, and it increases the risk of several types of cancer, gallbladder disease, musculoskeletal disorders and respiratory symptoms. In some populations, the metabolic consequences of weight gain start even at modest levels of overweight. The costs attributable to obesity are high not only in terms of obesity's contribution to increased health care costs and premature death, particularly from co-morbid diseases, but also in view of related disabilities and diminished quality of life.

The prevalence of overweight and obesity is escalating rapidly worldwide. In many developing countries overweight and obesity co-exist with undernutrition. This presents a double burden for those countries and their efforts to combat both should be balanced carefully. There is an urgent need to prevent or reverse unhealthy trends in diet and physical activity patterns in developing countries.

Prevention of overweight and obesity should begin early in life. It should involve the development and maintenance of life-long healthy eating and physical activity patterns. In adults, the prevention of overweight should include efforts to prevent further weight gain even when BMI is still in the acceptable range. Healthy lifestyles, including balanced diets of lower energy density (increased vegetables, fruits, grains and cereals) with increased levels of physical activity (such as walking) and reduction in <u>sedentary behavior</u>, should be promoted. Prevention is not just the responsibility of individuals but requires <u>structural changes in societies.</u>　　［出典 Quantum URL; H. p.251, l. 3〜17, l. 28〜36］

Notes　BMI：body mass index, 体格指数　squared：二乗の　morbidity：罹患率　mortality：死亡率　determinant：決定因子　NCD：non-communicable disease, 非伝染性疾患　NIDDM：non-insulin-dependent diabetes mellitus, 成人型インスリン非依存性糖尿病　CHD：coronary heart disease, 冠動脈性心臓病　gallbladder disease：胆道疾患　musculoskeletal：筋骨格系の　The costs attributable to obesity：肥満に起因する（疾病）負担は…　co-morbid：共存症　diminish：減少させる　prevalence：有病率　undernutrition：栄養不良　combat：闘う　reverse：方向転換させる　sedentary behavior：じっとして身体を動かすことの少ない過ごし方　structural change in societies：社会構造の改革

■ Post-reading activities

1. 次の英文を読んで正しいものにはTを，間違っているもにはFを（　　）に記入しなさい．

　(1) The BMI is obtained by multiplying the weight in kilograms by height measured in meters, squared (W/H^2).　(　)

　(2) People with BMIs of 22-25, men and women alike, are most likely to develop diseases and die early.　(　)

　(3) Obesity is a hereditary disease, so it cannot be prevented.　(　)

　(4) Obesity may cause lowered quality of life.　(　)

　(5) Being too heavy does not necessarily mean being unhealthy.　(　)

　(6) The prevalence of overweight is seen only in developed countries.　(　)

　(7) A population under the burden of undernutrition cannot be overweight.　(　)

　(8) In adults, prevention of overweight should be started only when the BMI is beyond the acceptable range.　(　)

　(9) Both individuals and societies are responsible for prevention of obesity.　(　)

(10) If you have a sedentary lifestyle, you need exercise. (   )

2. 文中でHealthy lifestyleとして，具体的にあげている3つの要件を書きなさい．
   (1)
   (2)
   (3)

3. "sedentary behavior" とはどんな行動でしょうか．あてはまるものに✓印を記入しなさい．
   (　) TV-watching　　(　) skiing　　(　) computer programming
   (　) playing golf　　(　) reading　　(　) fishing
   (　) mountain climbing　　　　　(　) jogging
   (　) writing out a homework　　(　) roller-blading
   (　) playing computer games　　(　) e-mailing
   (　) listening to music

4. Section IのPre-reading activitiesに登場した4人と，あなたのBMIの値を計算して記入しなさい．

   Yukiko's BMI　_____
   Mari's BMI　_____
   Koichi's BMI　_____
   Kazuo's BMI　_____
   Your BMI　_____

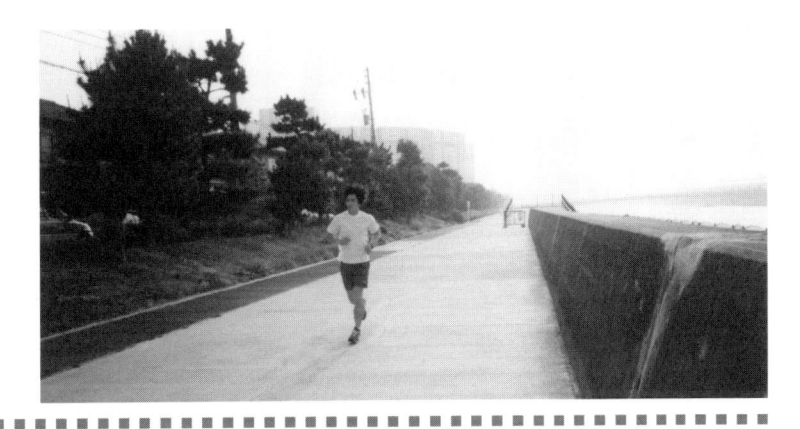

6：Obesity

やせていても，もっとやせたい若い女性
太っていても，平気な男性

体型を示す体格指数は次の公式で求められます．

$$BMI = [(体重kg)/(身長m)^2]$$

日本人のBMI判定では，＜18.5が「やせ」，18.5≦～＜25を「正常」，25≦を「肥満」としています．ところが，下の表のように現実には標準（BMI＝22）よりやせ気味の若い女性（15歳～19歳）にやせ願望のあることがわかります．

これに反して，男性は肥満であっても，そのうちの40％以上が，とくに体重コントロールを心掛けていません．

	年齢	15～19	20～29	30～39	40～49	50～59	60～69	70～
男性	現実	61.8 (21.2)	65.6 (22.4)	68.8 (23.6)	67.2 (23.7)	64.7 (23.6)	61.9 (23.5)	57.1 (22.4)
	理想	61.0 (20.7)	63.1 (21.5)	64.5 (22.0)	63.5 (22.2)	62.0 (22.4)	59.9 (22.5)	57.0 (22.1)
女性	現実	51.2 (20.6)	51.4 (20.6)	53.4 (21.6)	54.7 (22.7)	54.3 (23.3)	53.2 (23.7)	48.9 (23.0)
	理想	46.6 (18.7)	47.7 (19.1)	49.0 (19.7)	50.0 (20.6)	50.1 (21.3)	49.8 (21.8)	47.5 (21.9)

現実の体重と理想の体重
体重はkg，（ ）はBMI．
資料：厚生省「平成10年国民栄養調査結果の概要」

Chapter 7 Exercise

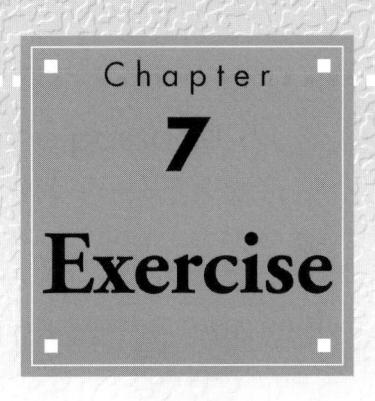

運動

I. Physical Activity and the Use of Calories

身体活動とエネルギー消費

FACTS

A person loses 25% of his or her lean body mass and 75% of his or her fat when losing weight through calorie reduction alone. In combination with physical activity, the loss in body fat is 98%.

■ Pre-reading activities

1. 次の質問に英語で答えて，自分の運動量をチェックしてみましょう．
   (1) How many hours do you exercise a week?
   (2) Do you like to stay in your room and watch TV for many hours?
   (3) Do you usually take the bus from the station to school?
   (4) Would you rather drive with your friends than play soccer or baseball on weekends?
   (5) Are you a member of a fitness club?

2. 次の表はいろいろな身体活動のカロリー（エネルギー）消費と，からだへの効果を比べたものです．表を見て，次の質問に英語で答えなさい．
   (1) What activity consumes the highest energy per 20 minutes?

7 : Exercise

	A	B	C	D
Easy walking	60	□	□	□
Light housework	90	□	□□	□□
Light gardening	90	□	□□	□□
Golf	90	□	□□	□
Brisk walking	100	□□	□	□□
Badminton	115	□□	□□□	□□
Gymnastics	140	□□	□□□□	□□
Heavy gardening	140	□□	□□□	□□□□
Dancing	160	□□	□□□	□
Easy jogging	160	□□□	□	□□
Tennis	160	□□□	□□□	□□
Skiing (downhill)	160	□□□	□□□	□□
Skiing (cross-country)	180	□□□□	□□□	□□
Football	180	□□□	□□□	□□
Handball	200	□□□	□□□	□□
Brisk jogging	210	□□□□	□□	□□
Bicycling	220	□□□□	□□	□□□
Swimming	240	□□□□	□□□□	□□□□

The fitness value of various activities
source : The American Medical Association, *Encyclopedia of Medicine*

A : Calories consumed in 20 minutes of activity   □□□□ : Excellent
B : Value in improving heart and lung fitness   □□□ : Good
C : Values in improving joint suppleness   □□   : Fair
D : Value in improving muscle power   □   : Minimal

(2) What activity burns off the lowest energy per 20 minutes?

(3) How many calories do you burn off by playing tennis for 40 minutes?

(4) What activities are recommended to improve joint suppleness?

(5) What activities improve your muscle power the most?

(6) What indoor sport is to be recommended to a person who wants to retain her joint suppleness by a moderate activity?

Read the passage

自分で進んで運動をすることを，生活の一部に組み入れることは，現代生活に欠かすことができません．運動するとなぜ健康に良いのでしょう．なぜ運動が必要なのでしょうか．

For most of history, diseases associated with diet were due to vitamin or mineral deficiencies, or simply to prolonged semi-starvation. In developed countries today, however, the main dietary threat to health is caused by excess.

While food is the body's energy source, people who engage in little exercise can easily become overweight by eating more than they "burn off" in physical activity. Regular exercise (at least three times a week) keeps the heart, lungs, muscles, and bones in good health and slows down the aging process. A person who is in good physical condition at the age of 60 can achieve up to 80 percent of the level of physical exertion that he or she could achieve in the mid-20s. Regular exercise improves the circulation in the heart and muscles and provides increased stamina. Exercise as simple as regular, brisk walking also maintains the density of bones, thus reducing the risk of developing osteoporosis ("thinning" and weakening of the bones) and fractures. A person who exercises regularly is less likely than a person who does not exercise sufficiently to have a heart attack or to die from a heart attack if one occurs.

[出典A. p.18, L11〜15, p.20, L3〜10, R1〜10]

Notes associated with〜：〜に起因する　deficiency：欠乏症　prolonged semi-starvation：長期にわたる半飢餓状態　dietary threat：食生活に起因する健康を脅かすもの　excess：過食　circulation：循環　osteoporosis：骨粗鬆症　fracture：骨折

Post-reading activities

上記のpassageの内容を読み取って次の質問に答えなさい．（英語または日本語）

（1）昔の食生活上の問題点：

（2）現代の食生活上の問題点：

（3）肥満の起こるしくみ：

（4）規則的な運動の持つ病気予防の効果：

■ Read the passage

運動するとからだはどうなるのでしょうか．

Physical activity is defined as the state of being active, or energetic action or movement.

- Physical activity can increase the <u>basal metabolic rate</u>, which is the number of calories used by the body when it is at rest. The increase in basal metabolic rate is <u>approximately</u> 10%, and possibly lasts for as long as 48 hours after the completion of the activity.
- Physical activity helps in the utilization of calories. The number of calories used is dependent on the type and <u>intensity</u> of the activity, and on the body weight of the person performing the physical activity.
- Physical activity assists in reducing the <u>appetite</u>.
- For the purpose of weight loss, physical activity can reduce <u>body fat</u> and is more <u>beneficial</u> in combination with reduced intake of calories.
- Physical activity also helps in the maintenance and control of weight.

［出典URL③］

運動によるカロリー消費量は，時間，体重，ペースによって決まります．

The following are some <u>variables</u> when physical activity and calorie expenditure is considered:

- Time: The amount of time spent on physical activity affects the amount of calories that will be expended. For example, walking for 45 minutes will burn more calories than walking for 20 minutes.
- Weight: The body weight of a person doing the physical activity also impacts the amount of calories used. For example, a 250-<u>pound</u> person will expend more energy walking for 30 minutes than a 185-pound person.
- Pace: The rate at which a person performs the physical activity will

also affect the amount of calories used. For example, walking 3 miles per hour will burn more calories than walking 1.5 miles per hour.

[出典 URL ③]

Notes basal metabolic rate：基礎代謝率 approximately：約 intensity：密度 appetite：食欲 body fat：体脂肪 beneficial：有益な variable：(変数)要因 pound：1 pound ＝ 0.45 kg mile：1 mile ＝ 1.61 km

▍Post-reading activities

次の英文のうち，正しいものにはT，間違っているもにはFを(　)に記入しなさい．

(1) The basal metabolic rate is the number of calories used by the body when it is in motion. (　)

(2) Regardless of the type of body, an individual can utilize a certain number of calories through physical activity. (　)

(3) Your appetite is enhanced by physical activity. (　)

(4) You can lose twice as much weight by walking double the distance. (　)

(5) A heavy person may expend more calories than a lighter person. (　)

食べても太らない人，太る人──「倹約遺伝子」のはなし

人間のからだは，タンパク質や炭水化物を貯蔵することができないので，余分なものは，脂肪にかえて貯蔵します．脂肪細胞ができたり，肥大化するときに働く遺伝子は，食べたものを脂肪として効率良く貯え，残りのわずかなエネルギーでからだを動かすことができるような働きがあります．この「倹約遺伝子」は日本人には欧米人よりも多いのです．

でも欧米人ほど肥満者の割合が目立たないのはなぜ？

それは，もともと日本人にはインスリンを分泌する能力が低く，余分な糖を脂肪に変えることができず，肥満に至る前に糖尿病になりやすいからなのです．

II. Guidelines for Exercise

よい運動のためのガイドライン

FACTS

More than 70% of men in their 30s and 40s feel that they need to get more exercise. More than 80% of women in their 20s and 30s feel the same need.

Pre-reading activities

健康維持を目的とする運動として適切と思うものを選びなさい．

weight lifting   archery   jogging   roller skating
cross-country skiing   bowling   boxing   walking
handball   cycling   swimming

Read the passage

Guidelines for exercise include:

- If you are just starting an exercise program and have any health concerns (such as obesity), have your doctor conduct an exercise tolerance test to help you establish limits for your exercise program.
- Begin gradually (perhaps with brisk walking) and don't expect to "get into shape" overnight. Your fitness should start to improve within 3 months with consistent effort.
- You should be able to carry on a conversation while you are exercising. At the same time, you typically should work hard enough to sweat during each exercise period.
- In order to become fit, plan an exercise routine that will last 20 to 30 minutes at least 3 days a week. Include stretching before and after your exercise. This will help avoid injury. Remember to start slowly and listen to your body's pain messages. If it hurts, then you have

probably overdone it.
- While exercises such as weight lifting provide strength to the muscles, they do little for the fitness of the heart. <u>Aerobic exercises</u> strengthen the heart and lungs and should be part of the fitness routine. Examples of good aerobic exercises include: walking, running, jogging, swimming, cross-country skiing, rowing, rope skipping, dancing, racket sports, and cycling.
- The <u>duration</u> of your exercise routine should be at least 20 to 30 minutes, and for more dramatic fitness results 45 to 50 minutes. In addition, remember that aerobic exercise can't be "start and stop"—it must be <u>sustained</u> for at least a 10- to 12-minute period.
- Adjustments in exercise programs need to be made for children, pregnant women, obese adults, elderly people, disabled people, and heart-attack survivors. Programs should also be modified for high <u>altitudes</u> and extreme heat or cold conditions.
- Use good equipment (especially good shoes) for your fitness program and do some research into a new type of activity before <u>launching</u> a program.
- No exercise program ever goes smoothly. There may be <u>setbacks</u> (such as illness or injury), but these should not change your overall program. If necessary, <u>substitute</u> one exercise activity <u>for</u> another (for example, switch from running to swimming). If you do have a setback, don't start immediately at your previous level of activity. You should take about as long to get back to your previous level of activity as the time you were out of action.
- Exercise can be fun even though it may not seem fun at first. Don't be afraid to vary both the duration and type of exercise activity if your present one is getting boring.　　　　　　　　　　　　［出典 URL ④］

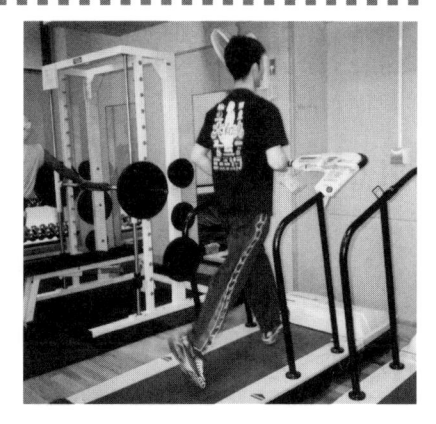

Notes　exercise tolerance：運動耐性限度(運動量の最大限界)　typically：普通は，通常は
routine：つねにおこなう決まった(運動)　aerobic exercise：有酸素運動　duration：継続時間

sustain：持続する　altitude：高度　launch：開始する　setback：後退，後戻り　substitute A for B：BとAを取替える

■■ Post-reading activities

1. 次の文章を完結させるのに最も適したものをa〜cの中から選びなさい．
   (1) You should consult your physician _____ .
      a.　if you have any health problems.
      b.　about a week after starting your exercise program.
      c.　before starting an exercise program.
   (2) Your fitness should start to improve within _____ .
      a.　four months
      b.　three months with consistent effort
      c.　eight weeks
   (3) While you are exercising, you should be able to carry on _____ .
      a.　a conversation
      b.　a meeting
      c.　a music performance
   (4) Weight lifting may strengthen the muscles, but not _____ .
      a.　bones
      b.　the mind
      c.　the heart
   (5) Adjustment in exercise programs need to be made for certain groups of people such as children, pregnant women and _____ .
      a.　depressed people
      b.　heart-attack survivors
      c.　company employees
   (6) It is necessary to choose _____ .
      a.　good equipment
      b.　an experienced trainer
      c.　an expensive course

2. 次の質問に英語で答えなさい．
   (1) How long does it typically take for your fitness to start to improve?

(2) Why should you include stretching before and after you exercise?

(3) What kinds of exercises strengthen the heart and lungs?

(4) How long should your exercise routine last if you wish dramatic fitness results?

(5) When would you vary the duration and type of exercise activity?

Seven Factors of Physical Fitness

Flexibility is the ability to bend, twist, and stretch the joints.
Coordination is the ability of all the parts of the body to interact smoothly.
Equilibrium is the ability to balance yourself.
Agility is the ability to move quickly with grace.
Speed is the measure of how fast the body moves.
Strength is the level at which your muscles are able to resist forces.
Endurance is the body's ability to handle stress for an extended period of time.

[出典 I. p.30, lower part l. 1〜7]

Chapter 8
Disabilities

障害

I. Where There's a Will, There's a Way

意志あるところ，道あり

> In Denmark, there are technical aids for all purposes, including leisure activities and sports. Disabled people have a great influence on product design and some manufacture aids themselves.

■ Pre-reading activities

1. もしあなたが，突然，車椅子の生活を余儀無くされたら，どのように感じるでしょうか．あてはまるものすべてに，○をつけなさい．

    I do not know how to spend my time.
    I do not know how to have a relationship with the opposite sex.
    I feel difficulties in my daily life.
    I am determined to get on with my life.
    I will try anything I can.
    I feel depressed.
    I feel almost the same as I was before.
    I mourn over my great misfortunes.
    I envy everyone around me because they can walk around freely.
    I am angry against myself.

Notes   get on with：どんどん進む

2. (　)に入る最も適切な語をa〜dから選びなさい．

(1) He was (　) from the chest down because of falling from a tree.
　　a. cut　　b. shocked　　c. paralyzed　　d. broken

(2) He can't walk, so he uses a (　).
　　a. wheelchair　　b. stool　　c. rocking chair　　d. couch

(3) He broke his (　) when he had a traffic accident.
　　a. spine　　b. spirits　　c. stomach　　d. throat

(4) He was in (　) of butterflies.
　　a. following　　b. pursuit　　c. pastime　　d. way

▪ Read the passage

DenmarkのJes Kleinは10年前，木から落ちたことがもとで障害をもつようになりました．彼はその後どのように生きたでしょうか．

Ten years ago, Jes Klein fell from a tree and broke his spine at the third vertebra. He was paralysed from the chest down, a paraplegic, and has since used a wheelchair.

Jes, a young and active sportsman, was suddenly forced to change his whole way of life. He had to give up his job as a plumber, and with only two arms functioning and a reduced lung capacity, his physical capabilities were severely restricted.

"All of a sudden I had 24 hours a day to fill and I didn't know how to spend all this spare time or what my options were. And I also had to find out how to have a relationship with the opposite sex again." says Jes.

However, Jes Klein soon regained his spirits. After 12 months of rehabilitation, a trip to USA, and fiercely determined to get on with his life, Jes threw himself into one leisure pursuit after another.

Jes has been water-skiing and driven motorcross on four-wheeled motorcycles. He swims all winter and using his hands. He cycles long trips at a speed that many non-disabled persons would have difficulty keeping up with. Eighteen months after the accident Jes met a girl, who already had a daughter, and last year he became a father for the second time.

Spurred by the desire and ability to lead an active life, both at

8 : Disabilities

work and at home on as normal terms as possible, Jes now runs his own business. He manufactures and sells high-performance wheelchairs for active users. His target groups are disabled people who want to be able to manage more than shopping at the local supermarket.

[出典J. p.8, *l.* 1〜p.9, *l.* 5]

Notes　spine：背骨　vertebra：脊椎骨　paralyse：麻痺させる　paraplegic：対麻痺の（患者）　wheelchair：車椅子　plumber：鉛管工　opposite sex：異性　regain one's spirits：元気を回復する　pursuit：追求　spur：かりたてる

■ Post-reading activities

1. ＿＿＿に入る最も適切なものをa〜cから選びなさい.

    (1) Jes uses a wheelchair because ＿＿＿.
       a. he was paralysed from the chest down due to a broken spine
       b. he fell from a tree and broke his legs
       c. he fell from a tree and his arms were paralysed

    (2) Due to paraplegia, ＿＿＿.
       a. he became a plumber
       b. his way of life has been changed a little
       c. his physical capabilities have been severely restricted

    (3) All of a sudden, Jes had 24 hours a day to fill and ＿＿＿.
       a. he spent all this spare time in a good way
       b. he didn't know what to do
       c. he spent all this spare time finding out how to have a relationship with the opposite sex

    (4) After 12 months of rehabilitation and a trip to USA, ＿＿＿.
       a. Jes remained depressed
       b. Jes recovered from his depression
       c. Jes began to run his own business

    (5) Eighteen months after the accident, ＿＿＿.
       a. Jes met a girl who already had a daughter
       b. Jes got married
       c. Jes became a father

    (6) Jes now runs his own business and ＿＿＿.
       a. he makes and sells high-performance wheelchairs for shop-

ping at the local supermarket
b. he manufactures and sells water-skis and motorcycles
c. he makes and sells high-performance wheelchairs for active users

2. 以下の英文は，あなたが車椅子に乗っている人に出会ったときのエチケットです．読んで後の質問に英語で答えなさい．

Wheelchair Etiquette

1. Always ask the wheelchair user if he or she would like assistance before you help. Your help may not be needed or wanted.
2. Don't hang or lean on a person's wheelchair. It is part of the wheelchair user's personal space.
3. Speak directly to the person in the wheelchair, not to someone nearby as if the wheelchair user does not exist or is a mental <u>defective</u>.
4. If the conversation lasts more than a few minutes, consider sitting down or kneeling to get yourself on the same level as the wheelchair user.
5. Don't <u>demean</u> or <u>patronize</u> the wheelchair user by patting him or her on the head or shoulder.
6. Give clear directions, including distance, weather conditions and physical obstacles that may hinder the wheelchair user's travel.
7. Don't discourage children from asking questions about the wheelchair. Open communication helps overcome fear and misleading attitudes.
8. When a wheelchair user transfers out of the wheelchair to a chair, toilet, car or bed, do not move the wheelchair out of reaching distance.
9. It is OK to use expressions like "running along" when

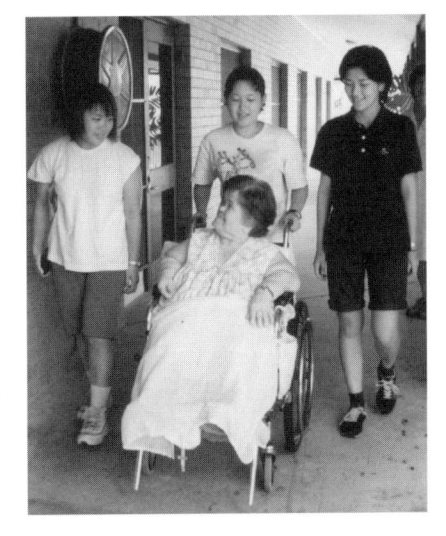

speaking to the wheelchair user. It is likely the wheelchair user expresses things the same way.

10. Be aware of the wheelchair user's capabilities. Some users can walk with assistance. They use wheelchairs to conserve energy and move about more quickly.

11. Don't classify people who use wheelchairs as sick. Wheelchairs are used for a variety of disabilities.

12. Don't assume that using a wheelchair is in itself a tragedy. It provides freedom and allows the user to move about independently.

[出典 K]

Notes defective：欠陥がある　demean：品位を傷つける　patronize：見下すような態度をとる

Questions

(1) What do you have to do before you help a wheelchair user?

(2) Whom do you have to talk to when you help a wheelchair user?

(3) What shouldn't you do when you help a wheelchair user?

(4) What do you have to consider if the conversation lasts more than a few minutes?

3. passageにでてきた表現を使って次の文を英訳しなさい．

   (1) 突然父が亡くなったので，どのようにして生活費を稼いだらよいのかわからなかった．　　know how to～：～の仕方を知っている

   (2) 1年間のオーストラリアでのホームステイの後，彼女は元気を取り戻した．
      regain one's spirits：元気を取り戻す

   (3) 彼は新聞を読むのに困難を感じた．
      have difficulty～ing：～するのに困難を感じる

II. Accessibility for All for the New Millennium

新ミレニアムに向けて，すべての人のために
アクセサビリティを

FACTS

The total number of people with disabilities in Japan is estimated at about 4.91 million, with about 2.95 million children (adults) with physical disabilities (1991 estimate), about 0.39 million children (adults) with mental retardation (1990 estimate) and about 1.57 million people with mental disorders (1993 estimate).
[Ministry of Health and Welfare]

Notes　mental retardation：精神遅滞　mental disorders：精神障害

Pre-reading activities

1. Aの表は「現在，どんな福祉サービスを必要としているか」という質問に対する身体障害者の人たちの答え，Bの表は同じ質問に対する精神障害者の人たちの答えです（複数回答）．2つの表と一致する英文をa〜eから選びなさい．

Table A
source：Survey on the Actual Status of Adults with Physical Disabilities, by the Ministry of Health and Welfare (1991)

Strengthening of income security measures such as pensions	40.7%
Alleviating medical care costs	20.3%
Strengthening of social welfare facilities	18.9%
Securing housing	13.0%
Equipping the environment and strengthening transportation systems	12.1%
Strengthening the assistance systems	11.6%
Implementing specialized rehabilitation training	10.0%

Notes　alleviate：軽減する

The understanding of others concerning people with disabilities	46.0%
A system that makes facilities available when needed	42.7%
Life after retirement	41.3%
Places to work	30.3%
Community facilities	22.5%

Table B
source : The Basic Survery of the Policy for the Welfare of Children (Adults) with Mental Retardation, by the Ministry of Health and Welfare (1990)

   a. Financial problems are the least concern of people with physical disabilities.
   b. The biggest concern of people with mental retardation is the understanding of others around them.
   c. More people with physical disabilities want to have social welfare facilities available than people with mental retardation.
   d. Basic requirements such as income security measures, medical care cost, and housing are the main concern of people with physical disabilities.
   e. People with mental retardation need places to work as well as people with physical disabilities.

2. （　）に入る最も適切な語をa〜dから選びなさい．
   (1) A lot of people come to the palace for the (　) of the Emperor's birthday.
      a. observatory   b. observance   c. observation
      d. preserve
   (2) (　) against anyone should not be allowed.
      a. Discrimination   b. Advantage   c. Privilege
      d. Differentiation
   (3) Freedom is a (　) of our civil, political, social and cultural rights.
      a. suggestion   b. demand   c. prerequisite
      d. supply
   (4) They have become ill as result of (　).
      a. welfare   b. disabilities   c. nutrition
      d. malnutrition

Read the passage

以下の英文は「国際障害者の日」における，国連事務総長のメッセージです．障害を持つ人たちにとってaccessibilityが大事だと主張しています．
accessibilityとはいったい何を意味しているのか，考えながら読みなさい．

The secretary general message on the international day of disabled persons

The theme for this year's observance of the International Day of Disabled Persons — accessibility — reminds us that for many people with disabilities, the lack of access to essential services remains a source of discrimination and lost opportunities.

For more than half a billion people in the world, accessibility can mean an education, a job and a community that would otherwise be denied for them. Accessibility is a prerequisite for disabled people to enjoy equal opportunities. It is a key to the exercise of their civil, political, social and cultural rights. This is a major concern of the United Nations, rooted in its founding principle of the equality of all human beings.

As computer-based communications and learning become more and more widespread, special needs must be taken into account. If they are not, the technological revolution will be lost on many talented people, and their contributions will be lost to the rest of us.

But we must not forget that 80 per cent of the world's disabled population lives in developing countries. Most of them have never used a phone, let alone a high-shaped computer. In many places, those who have become disabled as a result of malnutrition, land mine explosions or the acts of ruthless terrorists need access to water, food and health care as a matter of life and death. Meeting their basic needs must remain our highest priority.

Today, let us reaffirm our resolve to build truly accessible, caring and inclusive societies in the new Millennium.

[WHO. Press Release, SG/SM/7208, OBV/121]

Notes observance：祝うこと discrimination：差別 prerequisite：前提条件 malnutrition：栄養失調 land mine：地雷 ruthless：無慈悲な reaffirm：再び主張する resolve：決意 inclusive：包括的な

▐▐ Post-reading activities

1. 以下の質問に対する答えをa〜cから選びなさい．
   (1) What is accessibility?
       a. Accessibility means that many people with disabilities can use any transportation.
       b. Accessibility means that many people with disabilities can access to essential services from water to computer-based communication.
       c. Accessibility means that many people with disabilities can be accommodated into the facilities at any time.
   (2) Why is accessibility important for people with disabilities?
       a. Because computer-based communications and learning have become more and more widespread.
       b. Because accessibility brings money to people with disabilities.
       c. Because the lack of access to essential services leads to discrimination and lost opportunities.
   (3) Do the world's disabled population have access to essential services?
       a. Yes, most of them have access to various services.
       b. No, most of them have never used even a phone.
       c. Yes and No. Most of them have access to a phone but not to a computer-based communication.
   (4) What do those who have become disabled as a result of malnutrition, land mine explosion or the acts of ruthless terrorists need?
       a. They need access to basic services such as water, food and health care.
       b. They need computer-based communication and learning.
       c. They need civil, political, social and cultural rights.

2. passageにでてきた表現を使って次の文を英訳しなさい．

（1）この石碑は，ここで多くの人が地雷によって殺されたということを思いおこさせます． remind us that～：～ということを思いおこさせる

（2）携帯電話の使用はますます広がっています．
become more and more widespread：ますます広がって

（3）たいていの人はカロリーのとり過ぎの結果として肥満になります．
as a result of～：～の結果として

Chapter 9
Aging

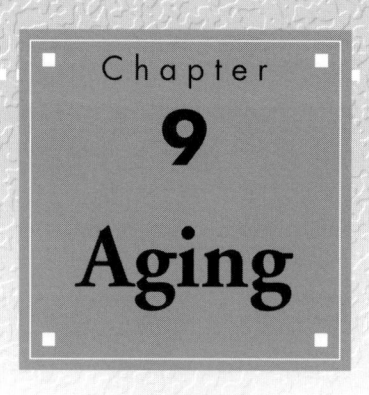

高齢化

I. Population Aging — A Public Challenge

高齢化―社会への挑戦

> **FACTS**
>
> By 2020 more than 1000 million people aged 60 years and older will be living in the world, more than 700 million of them in developing countries.

■ Pre-reading activities

1. グラフは上から各々1950年，2000年，2050年の東南アジアの年齢別，性別人口分布を表しています．(1)〜(4)の英文がグラフと一致していればTを，そうでなければFを（　　）に記入しなさい．

    (1) The population is aging gradually in Southeast Asia. （　）

    (2) In 1950, the number of children is more than that of the elderly. （　）

    (3) During the 100 years since 1950, both mortality and fertility have declined in Southeast Asia. （　）

    (4) People in 2050 will live longer than those in 1950. （　）

I. Population Aging

Percentage of total population. (both sexes)

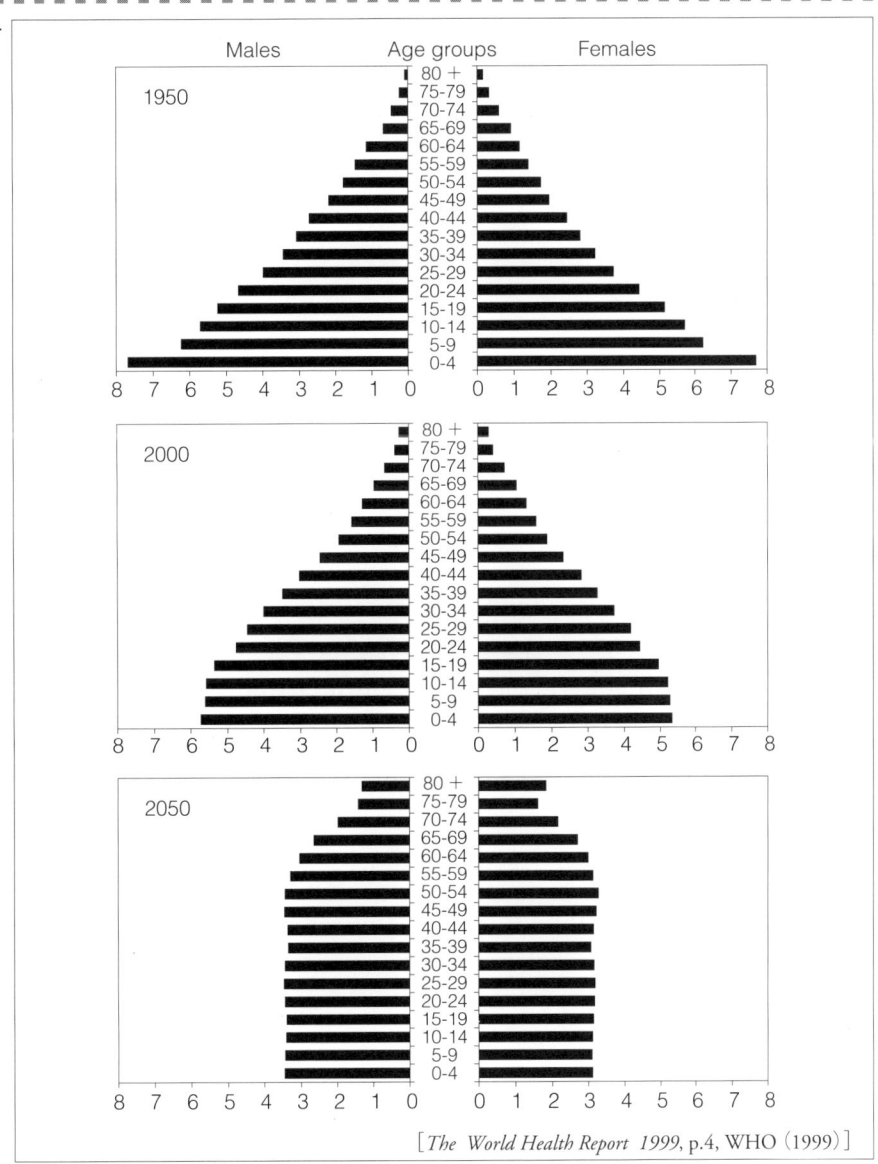

[Population pyramids for 1950, 2000, and 2050, by Males and Females across age groups from 0-4 to 80+]

[*The World Health Report 1999*, p.4, WHO (1999)]

2. (　　)の中に入る最も適切な語をa〜dから選びなさい．

(1) One of the (　　) features of the world population has been aging.

　　a. mathematics　　b. statistical　　c. demographic
　　d. democratic

(2) The decline of (　　) accelerates aging of the world population.

　　a. fertility　　b. mortality　　c. morbidity　　d. rate

(3) Technological (　　) in the field of medicine have contributed to aging of the world population.
   a. increase   b. breakthroughs   c. effects
   d. results

(4) Our life expectancy has increased due to medical (　　).
   a. exchange   b. interactions   c. help
   d. intervention

Read the passage

20世紀における世界の人口統計上の特徴は，高齢化です．けれども，高齢化も先進国と発展途上国とでは，事情が異なります．

One of the main features of the world population in the 20th century has been a considerable increase in the absolute and relative numbers of older people in both developed and developing countries. This phenomenon is referred to as "population aging". From a demographic point of view population aging is a result of both mortality and fertility: fewer children are born and more people reach old age.

In developed countries, population aging has evolved gradually as a result of an earlier decline in fertility and improving living standards for the majority of the population over a relatively long period of time after the industrial revolution. Technological breakthroughs in the field of medicine, including the development of new and effective drugs and vaccines, contributed to this process much later.

In developing countries, population aging is occurring more rapidly because of rapid fertility decline and an increasing life expectancy due to medical interventions based on the use of advanced technology and drugs. These interventions have provided effective means to treat and prevent many diseases that used to kill people prematurely. Also of importance is the fact that population aging in the developing world is accompanied by persistent poverty.

The rapidly growing absolute and relative number of older people in both developed and developing countries mean that more and more people will be entering the age when the risk of developing certain chronic and debilitating diseases is significantly higher. As such, population aging presents new and serious challenges for national and international public health.

By 2020, it is projected that three-quarters of all deaths in developing countries could be aging related. The largest share of these deaths will be caused by non-communicable diseases (NCDs), such as diseases of the circulatory system (CSDs), cancers and diabetes.

Many developing countries are already facing a double burden: the health problems of an aging population, and continuing high rates of communicable disease.

The emerging social and the public health consequences of aging, especially in developing countries, need to be taken very seriously. In the majority of these countries, poverty, lack of social security schemes, continuing urbanization and the growing participation of women in the workforce—all contribute to the erosion of traditional forms of care for older people.

Living longer is both an achievement and a perpetual challenge. Investing in health and promoting it throughout the life span is the only way to ensure that more people will reach old age in good health and capable of contributing to society intellectually, spiritually and physically.

[WHO. Fact Sheet N-135, Revised September 1998]

Notes phenomenon：現象 demographic：人口統計上の fertility：出生率 breakthrough：顕著な進歩 medical intervention：医療介入 prematurely：若くして persistent poverty：恒常的な貧困 chronic and debilitating disease：消耗性慢性疾患 project：推測する communicable disease：伝染性疾患 circulatory system：循環器系 diabetes：糖尿病 social security schemes：社会保障計画 erosion：崩壊 perpetual：とどまることのない life span：生涯

■ Post-reading activities

1. 以下の質問に対する最も適切な答えをa〜cから選びなさい．

　　(1) What phenomenon is referred to as "population aging"?

　　　　a. It is a considerable increase in the absolute numbers of adults

in both developed and developing countries.
  b. It is a considerable decrease in the absolute numbers of children in both developed and developing countries.
  c. It is a considerable increase in the old people in both developed and developing countries.
(2) What two demographic factors contribute to population aging?
  a. Morbidity and mortality.
  b. Mortality and fertility.
  c. Morbidity and fertility.
(3) What factors affected population aging in its earlier process in developed countries?
  a. An earlier decline in fertility and improved living standards for the majority of the population.
  b. Technological breakthroughs in the field of medicine, including the development of new and effective drugs and vaccines.
  c. Rapid fertility decline and an increasing life expectancy due to medical intervention.
(4) How is population aging occurring in developing countries?
  a. Population aging is occurring in the similar way as that in developed countries.
  b. Population aging is occurring more slowly.
  c. Population aging is occurring more rapidly.
(5) What factors contribute to the erosion of traditional forms of care for older people in the majority of developing countries?
  a. The increase of so-called nuclear families contributes to the erosion of traditional forms of care for older people.
  b. The increase of non-communicable diseases contributes to the erosion of traditional forms of care for older people.
  c. Poverty, lack of social security schemes, continuing urbanization and the growing participation of women in the workforce contribute to the erosion of traditional forms of care for older people.

2. passageにでてきた表現を使って次の文を英訳しなさい．

(1) 人口が都会に集中する現象を都市化と呼んでいます．
   refer to ~ : ~と呼ぶ

(2) 人口統計上のデータに基づいて，その町は計画されました．
   based on ~ : ~に基づいて

(3) 働く女性の増加が出生率の低下の一因となっています．
   contribute to ~ : ~の一因となる

II. Adult Development and Aging

能力開発と高齢化

> Population aging is having profound effects on society. It is a quiet, almost unseen social revolution.

Pre-reading activities

1. 20世紀の平均寿命は驚異的に伸びました．表を見て質問に英語で答えなさい．

   (1) What country shows the most remarkable increase in life expectancy at birth?

   (2) What country shows the smallest increase in life expectancy at birth?

   (3) What country enjoys the longest life expectancy at birth?

   (4) What effects do you think this remarkable increase in life expectancy will have on the society?

9 : Aging

Country	Around 1910		1998	
	Males	Females	Males	Females
Australia	56	60	75	81
Chile	29	33	72	78
England and Wales	49	53	75	80
Italy	46	47	75	81
Japan	43	43	77	83
New Zealand	60	63	74	80
Norway	56	59	75	81
Sweden	57	59	76	81
United States	49	53	73	80

Life expectancy at birth, selected countries, around 1910 and in 1998

[*The World Health Report 1999*, p.2, WHO (1999)]

2. （　）に入る最も適切な語をa～dから選びなさい．

(1) The facilities where some older people live are referred to as (　).
　a. elderly's homes　b. nursing homes
　c. day-care center　d. nursery

(2) Older people who have difficulty living alone are often (　).
　a. institutionalized　b. accommodated　c. hospitalized
　d. cared

(3) Given demographic (　), the health insurance fees were raised.
　a. results　b. provisions　c. projections　d. effects

(4) People with disabilities (　) for their physical ability in the work place and perform well.
　a. contribute　b. attribute　c. work
　d. compensate

■ Read the passage

ここでは，アメリカにおける高齢化の現実をとりあげ，それに対してどのように対処すればよいかを提起した英文を読みます．

The oldest-old

　The oldest-old, those aged 80 and older, is the most rapidly growing segment of our society. This growth in the number of adults in the 80 and older category, the majority of whom are women, is perhaps the most dramatic and most problematic aspect of the demographic changes in the United States population.

One in four of the oldest-old is in a nursing home. Of the remaining 75% who are not institutionalized, 45% needs assistance in the performance of everyday activities. An estimate of 20 to 25% of the oldest-old suffers from Alzheimer's Disease. Moreover, there is convincing scientific evidence that even the healthy, productive members of this age group experience significant levels of decline in their ability to function adequately in everyday activities.

First, there are significant declines in cognitive functioning of older adults. Accompanying these cognitive changes are significant decreases in the quality of social support for oldest-old adults because of the decreasing number of family and friends in their social networks.

Finally, reduced psychological well-being may accompany the typical losses in this age group: losses in physical health, losses of social companions, and loss of economic security. This reduced functioning leads to greater societal costs, including the costs of long-term care and institutionalization. Moreover, institutionalization in this age group often exacerbates the problems of psychological functioning rather than reducing them.

[出典 URL ⑤]

The older adults and work

As our work force ages, we must begin to understand how to use older adults as an important human resource in order to maintain the vitality and productivity of our work force. Earlier this century, retirement lasted a few years prior to death. Today, it may represent as much as a third of one's life. It is clear that changing demographics will profoundly influence decisions to continue working. Indeed, lower birth rates in the latter part of this century may force baby boomers to remain in the work force long after they had expected to retire, due to limited number of younger workers to support retirees.

Given demographic projections, it is imperative that we capitalize on the resources of older workers. Not only would it be difficult for this country to afford to have one third of its adult population out of the work place, it is also a waste of human capital.

9 : Aging

Despite declines in some functions and in health, middle-aged and older adults frequently perform at high level in a wide variety of work settings. Psychologists are just beginning to understand how older adults compensate in the work place for cognitive, physical, and health-related decline, and continue to perform effectively. Psychologists are well positioned to address the issue of work and aging and to develop ways to maximize productivity and maintain work behaviors well into old age.

[出典URL⑥]

Notes　nursing home：老人ホーム　institutionalize：施設に収容する　Alzheimer's Disease：アルツハイマー病　cognitive functioning：認知能力　exacerbate：悪化させる　projections：予測　imperative：肝要である　capitalize on：利用する　human capital：人的資源　compensate：補う

■ Post-reading activities

1. 以下の英文がpassageの内容と一致していればTを, そうでなければFを(　　) に記入しなさい.

   (1) Society in the near future will need the human resource of older adults due to the limited number of younger workers. (　　)

   (2) Working older adults are those who maintain the level of their cognitive, physical, and health-related functions that they had when they were young. (　　)

   (3) The number of people in the 80 and older is equally distributed among men and women. (　　)

   (4) The healthy, productive members of the oldest old adults are able to maintain their ability to function adequately in everyday activities. (　　)

   (5) Institutionalization may exert an adverse effect on the psychological functioning of the oldest people. (　　)

2. passageにでてきた表現を使って次の文を英訳しなさい.

   (1) 睡眠は人生の約3分の1をも占めています.
   　　as much as～：～もの

(2) 会社の再建にあたっては，現在の従業員と設備を利用すべきである．
　　　capitalize on～：～を利用する

(3) 困難な状況にもかかわらず，彼らは最後までやりぬいた．
　　　despite～：～にもかかわらず

3. 相対的な高齢化の一因は出生率の低下です．グラフは1950年と1998年とにおける出生率を表しています．次の英文がグラフと一致すればTを，一致しなければFを（　）に記入しなさい．

(1) Africa had the highest fertility rate in 1950. (　)
(2) The Eastern Mediterranean had the highest fertility rate in 1998. (　)
(3) Europe had the lowest fertility rate in 1998. (　)
(4) In general, the fertility rate has been declining in the world. (　)
(5) In South-East Asia and the Western Pacific, the fertility rate has dramatically declined. (　)

Declines in fertility by WHO Region, 1950 and 1998

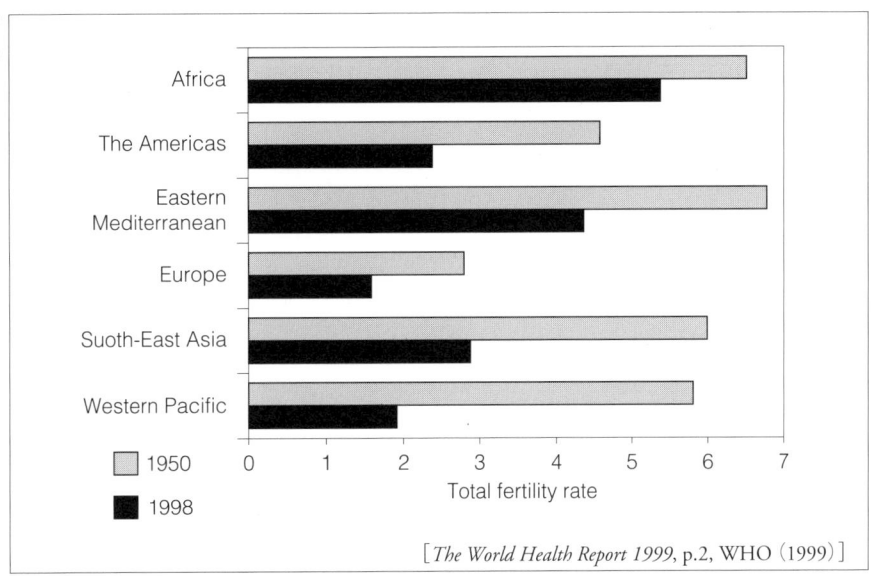

[*The World Health Report 1999*, p.2, WHO (1999)]

Chapter 10

Health Agenda for the 21st Century

21世紀への健康課題

I. Health Agenda for the 21st Century

21世紀への健康課題

Health and Human Rights

The enjoyment of the highest <u>attainable</u> standard of health is one of the <u>fundamental rights</u> of every human being without distinction of race, religion, political, economic or social conditions. (WHO Constitution)

Notes　attainable：入手可能な　fundamental rights：基本的人権

■ Pre-reading activities

1. グラフはWHOが，その加盟国（191か国）の1955年〜2025年までの健康改善目標としてかかげる3項目です．
   次の説明は，図のA，B，Cのどの項目に関連しているでしょうか．

   (1) <u>Infant mortality</u> has continued to decline in recent decades; it is expected that by 2025 there will be at least 151 countries (43% of global live births) with an infant mortality rate below 50 per 1000.

   (2) Life expectancy at birth has increased globally by 17 years, from 48 in 1955 to 65 in 1995, and is projected to reach a level of 73

I. Health Agenda for the 21st Century

Progress in achieving global targets for health for all by the year 2000

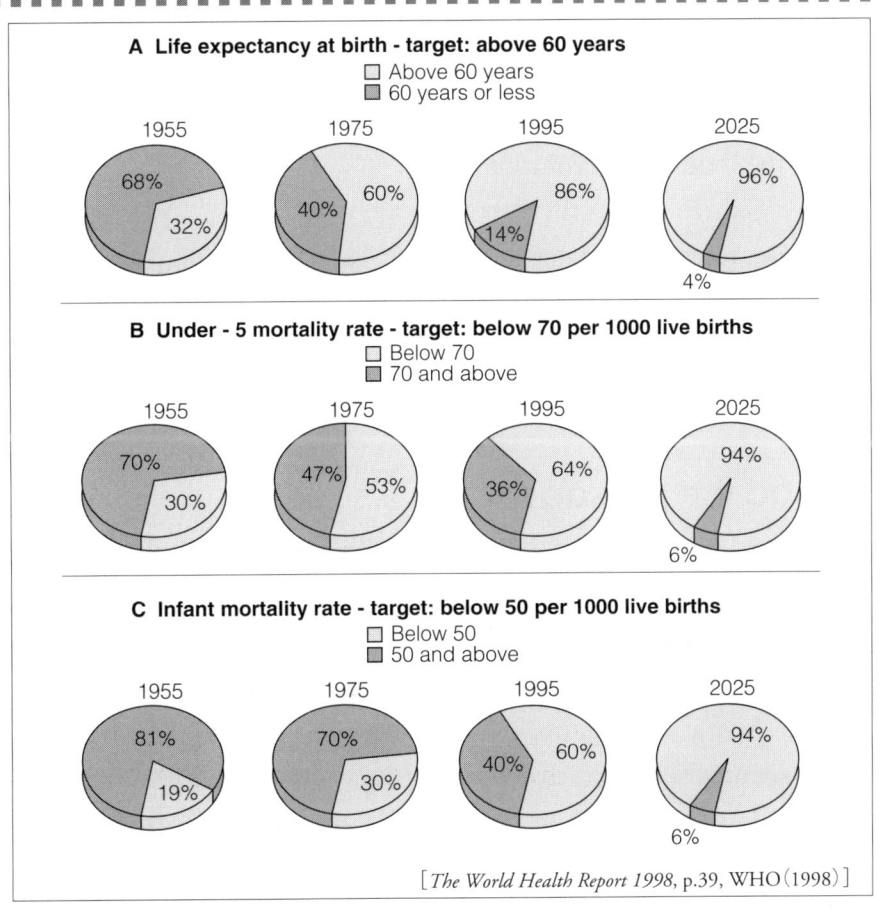

A Life expectancy at birth - target: above 60 years
☐ Above 60 years
■ 60 years or less

1955	1975	1995	2025
68% / 32%	40% / 60%	14% / 86%	4% / 96%

B Under - 5 mortality rate - target: below 70 per 1000 live births
☐ Below 70
■ 70 and above

1955	1975	1995	2025
70% / 30%	47% / 53%	36% / 64%	6% / 94%

C Infant mortality rate - target: below 50 per 1000 live births
☐ Below 50
■ 50 and above

1955	1975	1995	2025
81% / 19%	70% / 30%	40% / 60%	6% / 94%

[*The World Health Report 1998*, p.39, WHO (1998)]

years by 2025.

(3) In <u>the least developed countries</u>, the infant mortality rate changed only from 186 to 104 per 1000 between 1955 and 1995.

(4) The pace of progress in under-5 mortality reduction during 1975-1995 was not so fast as during 1955-1975.

(5) In all, more than 5 billion people now live in 120 countries where life expectancy at birth is above 60.

(6) The death rate per 100,000 population declined between 1955 and 1995 from 5280 to 1720 among children under 5.

Notes infant mortality：0歳児の死亡率 the least developed countries：発展途上国の中でも特に発展の遅れている国．国連の定義によれば "Those low-income countries that are suffering from long-term handicaps to growth, in particular, low levels of human resources development and/or structural weakness."

2. 次にあげる出来事のうち，20世紀に起こったものはどれでしょうか．（　　）に✓を記入しなさい．

(1) remarkable gains in health （　　）
(2) the Industrial Revolution （　　）
(3) rapid economic growth （　　）
(4) unprecedented scientific advances （　　）
(5) the World Wars （　　）
(6) eradication of smallpox （　　）
(7) invention of a vaccine against HIV/AIDS （　　）

Read the passage

次にあげるのは，WHOの最高責任者である事務局長の21世紀への展望を描いたメッセージです．

Message from the Director-General

　　The world enters the 21st century with hope but also with <u>uncertainty</u>. Remarkable gains in health, rapid economic growth and <u>unprecedented</u> scientific advance—all <u>legacies</u> of the 20th century—could lead us to a new era of human progress. But <u>darker legacies</u> bring uncertainty to this vision and demand redoubled <u>commitment</u>. <u>Regional conflicts</u> have replaced the global wars of the first half of the 20th century as a source of continued misery. Deep poverty remains all too <u>prevalent</u>. The <u>sustainability</u> of a healthy environment is still unproved. <u>The Universal Declaration of Human Rights</u>—now half a century old—is only a <u>tantalizing</u> promise for far too many of our fellow humans. The HIV/AIDS epidemic continues unchecked in much of the world, and it warns us against <u>complacency</u> about other, still unknown <u>microbial threats</u>.

　　With <u>vision</u>, commitment and successful leadership, the world could end the first decade of the 21st century with notable <u>accomplishments</u>. Many of the world's poor people would no longer suffer today's burden of premature death and excessive disability, and poverty itself would thereby be much reduced. <u>Healthy life expectancy</u> would increase for all. Smoking and other risks to health would fade in significance. The financial burdens of medical needs would be more fairly shared, leaving no household without access to care or exposed to economic ruin as a result of health expenditure. And health systems would respond with greater <u>compassion</u>, quality and efficiency to the increasingly <u>diverse</u> demands they face. Progress in the 20 th century points to the real opportunity for reaching these goals.

[出典 L. p. vii, l. 8〜21, l. 26〜35]

Notes   uncertainty：不確実性　unprecedented：いまだかつてなかったような　legacy：遺産　darker legacies：負の遺産　commitment：取り組み　regional conflicts：地域紛争　prevalent：はびこっている　sustainability：持続可能性　The Universal Declaration of Human Rights：世界人権宣言　tantalizing：簡単そうに見えるが，実際はなかなか実現困難な　complacency：油断　microbial threats：微生物の脅威　vision：未来設計　accomplishment：成果　healthy life expectancy：健康寿命 (p.9, DALEの項参照)　compassion：思いやり　diverse：多様な

■■Post-reading activities

　このpassageは２つのパラグラフ（paragraph）から構成されています．それぞれのパラグラフについて内容を読み取りましょう．

1. １番目のパラグラフの内容が，一文の中に要約されているのは，次のどの文ですか．
    (1) The world enters the 21st century with hope but also with uncertainty.
    (2) But darker legacies bring uncertainty to this vision.
    (3) The sustainability of a healthy environment is still unproved.
    (4) Deep poverty remains all too prevalent.

2. １番目のパラグラフの中で，"darker legacies"としてあげられている５つの項目を書き出しなさい．
    (1)
    (2)
    (3)
    (4)
    (5)

3. 2番目のパラグラフで，21世紀に達成可能な目標としてあげられている5つの項目を書き出しなさい．
   (1)
   (2)
   (3)
   (4)
   (5)

「健康日本21」は，厚生省による21世紀の日本人の健康目標です．表は2010年までの達成目標の一部です．あなたの現状はどうなっているでしょうか．

「健康日本21」のかかげる目標

	現 状	目 標
未成年の喫煙	中1 男 7.5％ 女 3.8％ 高1 男 36.9％ 女 15.6％	いずれも0
肥満者(BMI≧25)	20〜60歳代 男 24.3％ 20〜60歳代 女 25.2％	15％以下 20％以下
歩数	男 8,202歩 女 7,282歩	9,200歩 8,300歩
1日当たりの食塩摂取量	13.5 g	10 g
1日当たりの野菜の平均摂取量	292 g	350 g以上
1日の食事で果物を食べる人	29.3％	60％以上
健康診断を受ける人	4,573万人	5割以上増加

II. Global Health Care System
— Health in the Digital Age

デジタル時代がもたらすもの

> The health of all peoples is fundamental to the attainment of peace and security. (Preamble to the Constitution)

Notes　preamble：前文　the Constitution：WHO憲章

Pre-reading activities

1. 次の病気や障害のうち，現在，一般的に unavoidable disease and disability とされているのはどれでしょうか．また，avoidable disease and disability はどれですか．

| traffic accident   poliomyelitis   tuberculosis   water-born diseases |
| cancer   diabetes mellitus   undernutrition   hypertension   leukemia |

Avoidable：

Unavoidable：

2. WHO の提唱する "Health for All" とは何を意味するか，次の英文を読みましょう．

Health for All

"Health for All" does not mean an end to disease and disability, or that doctors and nurses will care for everyone. It means that resources for health are evenly distributed and that essential health care is accessible to everyone. It means that health begins at home, in schools, and at the workplace, and that people use approaches for preventing illness and <u>alleviating</u> unavoidable disease and disability.

It means that people <u>recognize</u> that ill-health is not <u>inevitable</u> and that they can <u>shape</u> their own lives and the lives of their families, free from the avoidable burden of disease.　　　　　　　　　　　[WHO]

Notes　alleviating：苦痛を軽減する　recognize：認識する　inevitable：仕方がない，まぬがれることのできない　shape：形成する

Read the passage

Health for All を実現するための手段の一つに，情報技術の発達により可能になった "telemedicine" ―「遠隔医療」があります．

What is telemedicine?

<u>Telemedicine</u> is the practice of medical care using <u>interactive</u> audio, visual and data communications; this includes medical care delivery, consultation, <u>diagnosis</u> and treatment, as well as education and

the transfer of medical data.

Telemedicine is, technically, the use of any electric signal to transmit medical information. The range of uses is almost unlimited.

The rapid growth of telemedicine is a worldwide phenomenon. However, the growth of telemedicine has not been uniform, either geographically or across all types of health care services. A nationalized health care system combined with the presence of many remote communities have spurred many countries in the world into investing in telemedical systems linking hospital centers with smaller clinics in remote villages. Scandinavia, especially Norway, was one of the first areas to widely deploy telemedicine. Extensive projects using telemedicine to deliver health care have been established in France, the United Kingdom, Japan, Australia, and Canada. Many other countries are in the process of setting up their own programs. Lesser-developed nations have shown a keen interest in using telemedicine to improve access to high quality health care but often lack both a telecommunications infrastructure or the resources to pay for such access.

The benefit of telemedicine is that the best medical resources can be delivered to a remote site anywhere in the world through the information superhighway. Telemedicine has the potential to provide great advances in the medical field. Instant access to information and the creation of an international medical society could create a new era where medicine is more efficient, more accurate, and more available to all.

[出典 URL ⑦]

Notes　telemedicine：遠隔医療，コンピューテイング遠隔治療　interactive：双方向の　diagnosis：診断　transfer：伝送　nationalized health care system：国民皆健康保険制度　remote communities：へき地の町村　spur：急がせる，推進させる，せきたてる　invest：投資する　deploy：展開させる　infrastructure：社会基盤　resources：資源，財源　the information superhighway：情報の高速道路（インターネットを指す）　potential：可能性

Post-reading activities

1. _____ に入る最も適切なものをa〜cから選びなさい．

    (1) The beauty of telemedicine is that the best medical resources can be delivered to a remote site anywhere in the world through ___.
       a. air transportation
       b. the information superhighway
       c. the fastest vehicle

    (2) The rapid growth of telemedicine is a _____ phenomenon.
       a. regional
       b. worldwide
       c. localized

    (3) Extensive projects using telemedicine to deliver health care have been established in _____.
       a. France, the United Kingdom, Japan, Australia, and Canada
       b. Norway, Switzerland, and the United States.
       c. France, the United States, Japan, Austria, and Canada

    (4) Telemedicine has the _____ to provide great advances in the medical field.
       a. ability
       b. capacity
       c. potential

    (5) Instant access to information and the creation of an international medical society could create a new era where medicine is more efficient, more accurate, and _____.
       a. more available to all
       b. less expensive
       c. more extensive

2. 次の質問に英語で答えなさい．

    (1) In nationalized telemedicine systems, what are hospital centers typically linked with?

(2) What country in Scandinavia was one of the first areas to deploy telemedicine nationwide?

(3) What is the benefit of telemedicine?

(4) Do you think individuals who don't have means of access to the Internet could enjoy the same quality of medical service as those who do?

3. telemedicine の発達によって恩恵を受けると思われる人を選びなさい.
   (1) chronically ill people who cannot go out on their own
   (2) patients with acute medical problems and living in remote areas who need medical advice
   (3) healthy people living in an urban area with adequate health care institutions
   (4) obese people who want privacy in getting dietary advice for planning their weight loss program
   (5) smaller clinics which need a specialist's medical guidance

---

e-health とは？

　e-health の e- は，e-mail, e-commerce（電子取引）の e- と同じように，electronic の略号です．e-health は次のような意味をあらわします．

　"E-health is a catchall term for everything from telemedicine, in which a doctor uses telecommunications technology to provide remote health care, to consumer-oriented health Web sites and sophisticated online databases that could reduce medical errors." (Barbara Fedee, *The San Jose Mercury News*, 2000 による)

　自宅のコンピュータからインターネットで医療や健康に関する情報，サービスを簡単に，豊富に入手できる時代が目前に来ています．しかし，これにともなって，このようなインターネットが可能にする情報空間（cyberspace）に参入できる人と，主として経済的な理由から参入できない人との格差（digital divide）が社会的な問題となります．また，国際的には，この格差が "Health for All" の WHO の理想への大きな挑戦となることが予想されます．

著者紹介

阿部 祐子（あべ としこ）
  1960年　大阪外国語大学外国語学部英語学科卒業
  1994年　テンプル大学教育学部大学院修了（TESOL専攻）
  　　　　元神戸学院大学他 非常勤講師

正木 美知子（まさき みちこ）
  1973年　神戸大学文学部英米文学科卒業
  1995年　テンプル大学教育学部大学院修了（TESOL専攻）
  現　在　大阪国際大学 特任教授

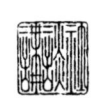

NDC 490　102 p　26 cm

英語で読む21世紀の健康
2000年　9月10日　第1刷発行
2017年　3月10日　第7刷発行

著　者　阿部祐子・正木美知子
発行者　鈴木　哲
発行所　株式会社　講談社
　　　　〒112-8001　東京都文京区音羽2-12-21
　　　　　　販　売　(03)5395-4415
　　　　　　業　務　(03)5395-3615
編　集　株式会社　講談社サイエンティフィク
　　　　代表　矢吹俊吉
　　　　〒162-0825　東京都新宿区神楽坂2-14　ノービィビル
　　　　　　編　集　(03)3235-3701
印刷所　株式会社双文社印刷・半七写真印刷工業株式会社
製本所　株式会社国宝社

落丁本・乱丁本は、購入書店名を明記のうえ、講談社業務宛にお送り下さい．送料小社負担にてお取替えします．なお、この本の内容についてのお問い合わせは講談社サイエンティフィク宛にお願いいたします．
定価はカバーに表示してあります．

© T. Abe and M. Masaki, 2000
本書のコピー、スキャン、デジタル化等の無断複製は著作権法上での例外を除き禁じられています．本書を代行業者等の第三者に依頼してスキャンやデジタル化することはたとえ個人や家庭内の利用でも著作権法違反です．

JCOPY 〈(社)出版者著作権管理機構 委託出版物〉
複写される場合は、その都度事前に(社)出版者著作権管理機構（電話 03-3513-6969, FAX 03-3513-6979, e-mail: info@jcopy.or.jp）の許諾を得てください．

Printed in Japan

ISBN4-06-153664-8

講談社の自然科学書

はじめての臨床栄養英語
清水 雅子／J.パトリック バロン・著
B5・121頁・本体2,300円（税別）

栄養管理を必要とする疾患を中心に、平易な英文で、組織・器官の名称、病気の概要、診断基準、食事療法、薬物療法を学ぶこれまでにない教科書。病院臨地実習やゼミで必須となる基本英語を集約。大学院受験にも役立つ。

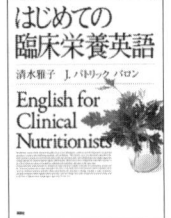

ニュースで読む医療英語
川越 栄子・編著　森 茂／田中 芳文／名木田 恵理子／大下 晴美・著
CD付き
B5・110頁・本体2,800円（税別）

医療・看護のためのやさしい英語テキスト。一般向けのわかりやすい医療ニュースを題材にするから、入門レベルの読者でもすらすら読める。ネイティブ読み上げCD付きでリスニングもバッチリ！

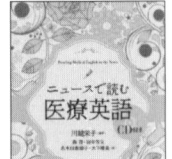

はじめての栄養英語
清水 雅子・著
B5・108頁・本体1,800円（税別）

やさしい英文で初学者でも栄養英語に親しめるよう工夫されたテキスト。栄養素、代謝、解剖生理、消化吸収、食品添加物、食物アレルギーなどを、やさしく短い英文でとりあげた。

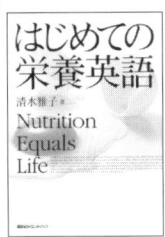

臨床心理士指定大学院対策
鉄則10＆キーワード100　心理英語編
河合塾KALS・監修
木澤 利英子・著
A5・237頁・本体2,500円（税別）

臨床心理士指定大学院合格へのキーワード100と英文読解の鉄則10を網羅。「ヒルガードの心理学」を題材に論述問題に慣れよう。入試傾向分析や関連用語も充実！

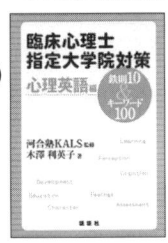

Let's Study English!
Health and Nutrition
英語で読む健康と栄養
横尾 信男・編著
A5・94頁・本体1,500円（税別）

栄養系学生のための教養課程英語テキスト。健康な食生活に必要な知識（栄養素やその摂取法、病気にならない食生活・エクササイズ、酒やタバコの害、食中毒、ストレス解消など）を幅広く学べるよう編集。

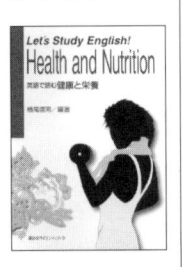

耳から学ぶ楽しいナース英語
中西 睦子・監修　野口 ジュディー／川越 栄子／仁平 雅子・著
CD付き
B5・110頁・本体3,400円（税別）

CDを聞きながら学ぶ看護英語の決定版。国際化時代の医療現場では英語は不可欠の時代、聞きとれること話せることは必須要素。「どうかしましたか」「どのように痛みますか」こんな会話が話せるようになる1冊。CD付き。

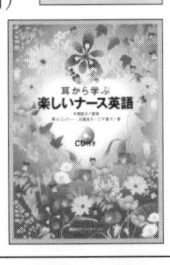

入門薬学英語
野口 ジュディー／神前 陽子／籠田 智美／山口 秀明・著
CD付き
B5・124頁・本体2,800円（税別）

多様な文例とCDで身につく「読む」「聞く」英語力。教養英語ではなく、薬学専門で使える英語の力を養う。医療関係の一般用語と専門用語の単語を学ぶことから始め、多様な文例で文体を覚え、英文に慣れることを狙う。CD付き。

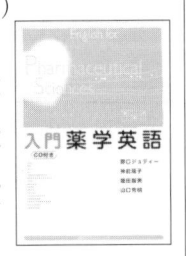

医療薬学英語
野口 ジュディー／神前 陽子／三木 知博／籠田 智美／山口 秀明・著
B5・142頁・本体3,000円（税別）

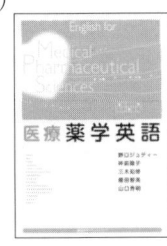

医療の英単語がわかり、英文速読の力がつく。医療現場でも多用される英語、そこでのコミュニケーション力向上を目的に医療関係の単語を多数収載。また、英文を「読める」から「速読できる」に重点を置き実用性を志向。

表示価格は本体価格（税別）です。消費税が別に加算されます。　　「2017年2月20日現在」

講談社サイエンティフィク　http://www.kspub.co.jp/

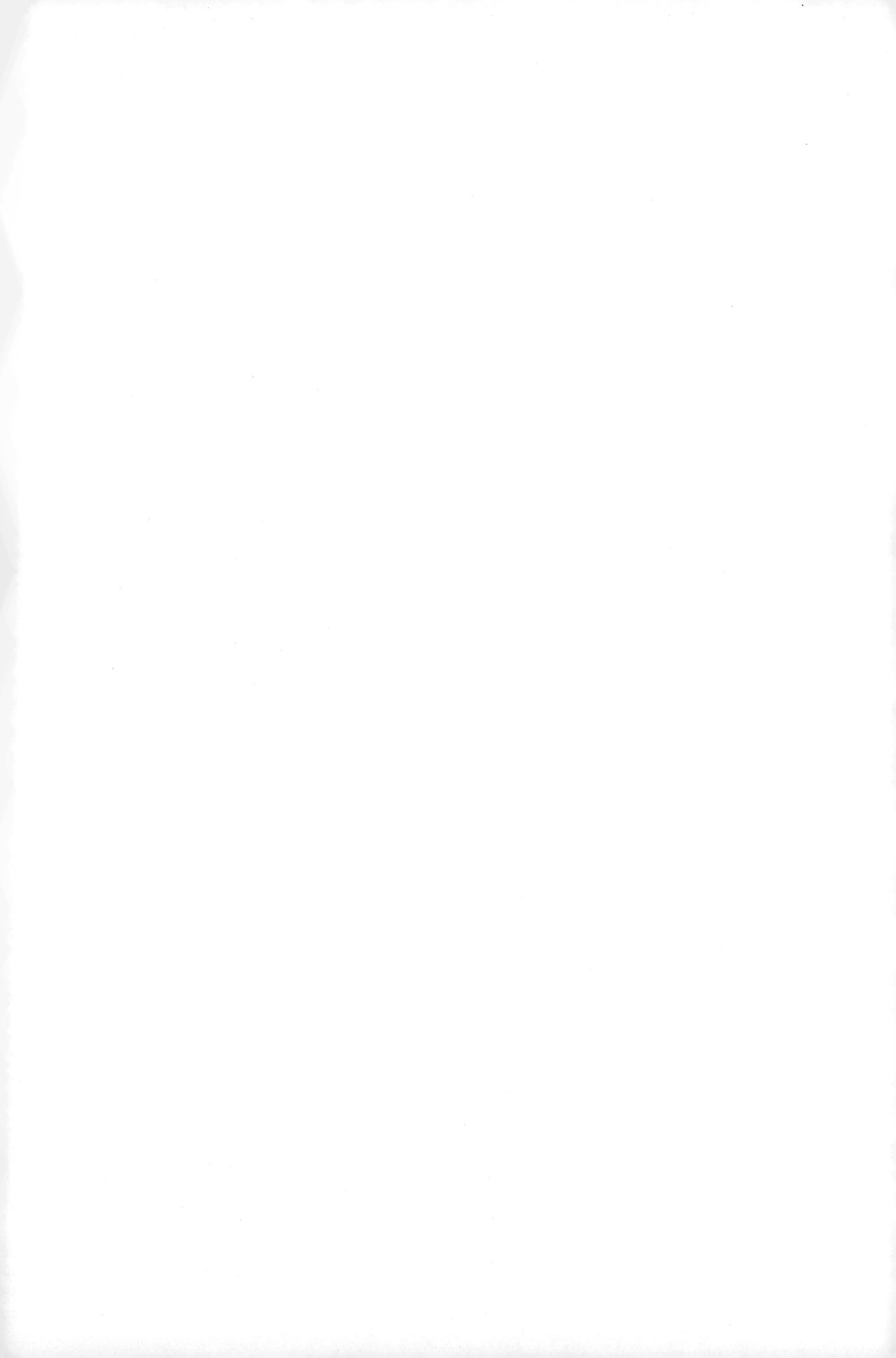